Recurrent First Trimester Pregnancy Loss

Editor

WILLIAM H. KUTTEH

OBSTETRICS AND GYNECOLOGY CLINICS OF NORTH AMERICA

www.obgyn.theclinics.com

Consulting Editor
WILLIAM F. RAYBURN

March 2014 • Volume 41 • Number 1

ELSEVIER

1600 John F. Kennedy Boulevard ● Suite 1800 ● Philadelphia, Pennsylvania, 19103-2899

http://www.theclinics.com

OBSTETRICS AND GYNECOLOGY CLINICS OF NORTH AMERICA Volume 41, Number 1
March 2014 ISSN 0889-8545, ISBN-13: 978-0-323-29024-1

Editor: Kerry Holland
Developmental Editor: Stephanie Carter

Obstetrics and Gynecology Clinics (ISSN 0889-8545) is published quarterly by Elsevier Inc., 360 Park Avenue South, New York, NY 10010-1710. Months of issue are March, June, September, and December. Periodicals postage paid at New York, NY, and additional mailing offices. Subscription price per year is $310.00 (US individuals), $545.00 (US institutions), $155.00 (US students), $370.00 (Canadian individuals), $688.00 (Canadian institutions), $225.00 (Canadian students), $450.00 (foreign individuals), $688.00 (foreign institutions), and $225.00 (foreign students). To receive student/resident rate, orders must be accompanied by name of affiliated institution, date of term, and the signature of program/residency coordinator on institution letterhead. Orders will be billed at individual rate until proof of status is received. Foreign air speed delivery is included in all *Clinics* subscription prices. All prices are subject to change without notice. POSTMASTER: Send address changes to *Obstetrics and Gynecology Clinics*, Elsevier Health Sciences Division, Subscription Customer Service, 3251 Riverport Lane, Maryland Heights, MO 63043. **Customer Service: Telephone: 1-800-654-2452 (U.S. and Canada); 314-447-8871 (outside U.S. and Canada). Fax: 314-447-8029. E-mail: journalscustomerservice-usa@elsevier.com (for print support); journalsonlinesupport-usa@elsevier.com (for online support).**

Reprints. For copies of 100 or more of articles in this publication, please contact the Commercial Reprints Department, Elsevier Inc., 360 Park Avenue South, New York, New York 10010-1710. Tel.: 212-633-3874; Fax: 212-633-3820; E-mail: reprints@elsevier.com.

Obstetrics and Gynecology Clinics of North America is also published in Spanish by McGraw-Hill Interamericana Editores S.A., P.O. Box 5-237, 06500, Mexico; in Portuguese by Reichmann and Affonso Editores, Rio de Janeiro, Brazil; and in Greek by Paschalidis Medical Publications, Athens, Greece.

Obstetrics and Gynecology Clinics of North America is covered in MEDLINE/PubMed (Index Medicus), Excerpta Medica, Current Concepts/Clinical Medicine, Science Citation Index, BIOSIS, CINAHL, and ISI/BIOMED.

Printed and bound by CPI Group (UK) Ltd, Croydon, CR0 4YY

Contributors

CONSULTING EDITOR

WILLIAM F. RAYBURN, MD, MBA
Professor and Chair, Department of Obstetrics and Gynecology; Associate Dean, Continuing Medical Education and Professional Development, University of New Mexico School of Medicine, Albuquerque, New Mexico

EDITOR

WILLIAM H. KUTTEH, MD, PhD, HCLD
Clinical Professor, Department of Obstetrics and Gynecology, Division of Reproductive Endocrinology and Infertility, Vanderbilt University School of Medicine, Nashville; Consulting Gynecologist, Department of Surgery, St. Jude Children's Research Hospital, Memphis; Director, Recurrent Pregnancy Loss Center, Managing Partner, Fertility Associates of Memphis, Memphis, Tennessee

AUTHORS

PAUL R. BREZINA, MD, MBA
Assistant Clinical Professor, Department of Obstetrics and Gynecology, Division of Reproductive Endocrinology and Infertility, Vanderbilt University School of Medicine, Nashville; Consulting Gynecologist, Department of Surgery, St. Jude Children's Research Hospital, Memphis; Director of Reproductive Genetics, Fertility Associates of Memphis, Memphis, Tennessee

OLE B. CHRISTIANSEN, MD, DMSc
Professor, Consultant in Department of Obstetrics and Gynecology, Fertility Clinic 4071, Copenhagen University Hospital, Copenhagen; Department of Obstetrics and Gynecology, Aalborg University Hospital, Aalborg, Denmark

WILLIAM B. DAVENPORT, MD
Department of Obstetrics and Gynecology, University of Vermont, Burlington, Vermont

FEROZA DAWOOD, MBChB, MRCOG, MD
Consultant in Obstetrics and Gynaecology, Department of Obstetrics, Liverpool Women's Hospital, Liverpool, United Kingdom

ROY G. FARQUHARSON, MD, FRCOG
Consultant in Gynaecology, Liverpool Women's Hospital, Liverpool, United Kingdom

MARIËTTE GODDIJN, MD, PhD
Department of Obstetrics and Gynaecology, Center for Reproductive Medicine, Academic Medical Center, Amsterdam, The Netherlands

CANDACE D. HINOTE, MD
MidSouth OB GYN, Memphis, Tennessee

CAROLYN R. JASLOW, PhD
Department of Biology, Rhodes College, Memphis, Tennessee

RAYMOND W. KE, MD, HCLD
Clinical Professor of Obstetrics and Gynecology, Vanderbilt University, Nashville; Chief, Assisted Reproduction, Fertility Associates of Memphis, Memphis, Tennessee

WILLIAM G. KEARNS, PhD
Associate Professor, Department of Gynecology and Obstetrics, Johns Hopkins Medical Institutions, Baltimore; Director, The Center for Preimplantation Genetics, LabCorp, Rockville, Maryland

WILLIAM H. KUTTEH, MD, PhD, HCLD
Clinical Professor, Department of Obstetrics and Gynecology, Division of Reproductive Endocrinology and Infertility, Vanderbilt University School of Medicine, Nashville; Consulting Gynecologist, Department of Surgery, St. Jude Children's Research Hospital, Memphis; Director, Recurrent Pregnancy Loss Center, Managing Partner, Fertility Associates of Memphis, Memphis, Tennessee

KELLY M. MCNAMEE, MBChB(Hon)
Obstetric and Gynaecology Specialist Trainee, Department of Obstetrics, Liverpool Women's Hospital, Liverpool, United Kingdom

LESLEY REGAN, MBBS, MD, FRCOG
Professor, Department of Obstetrics and Gynaecology, St Mary's Campus, Imperial College London, London, United Kingdom

SOTIRIOS H. SARAVELOS, MBBS
Department of Obstetrics and Gynaecology, St Mary's Campus, Imperial College London, London, United Kingdom

M.M.J. VAN DEN BERG, MD
Department of Obstetrics and Gynaecology, Center for Reproductive Medicine, Academic Medical Center, Amsterdam, The Netherlands

ROSA VISSENBERG, MD
Department of Obstetrics and Gynaecology, Center for Reproductive Medicine, Academic Medical Center, Amsterdam, The Netherlands

Contents

Foreword   ix

William F. Rayburn

Preface: Recurrent Pregnancy Loss   xi

William H. Kutteh

Classic and Cutting-Edge Strategies for the Management of Early Pregnancy Loss   1

Paul R. Brezina and William H. Kutteh

> There are few conditions in medicine associated with more heartache to patients than recurrent pregnancy loss (RPL). The management of early RPL is a formidable clinical challenge for physicians. Great strides have been made in characterizing the incidence and diversity of this heterogeneous disorder and a definite cause of pregnancy loss can be established in more than half of couples after a thorough evaluation. In this review, current data are evaluated and a clear roadmap is provided for the evaluation and treatment of RPL.

Research Methodology in Recurrent Pregnancy Loss   19

Ole B. Christiansen

> The aim of this article is to highlight pitfalls in research methodology that may explain why studies in recurrent pregnancy loss (RPL) often provide very divergent results. It is hoped that insight into this issue will help clinicians decide which published studies are the most valid. It may help researchers to eliminate methodological flaws in future studies, which will hopefully lead to some kind of agreement about the usefulness of diagnostic tests and treatments in RPL.

The Evolving Role of Genetics in Reproductive Medicine   41

Paul R. Brezina and William G. Kearns

> As medicine has evolved over the last century, medical genetics has grown from nonexistence to one of the most visible aspects of how we understand and treat disease. This increased role of genetics within medicine will only increase in the coming years, and its role in reproductive medicine will be significant. Genetics has emerged as a primary focus of research with translational applications within reproductive medicine. The aim of this article is to outline the applications of genetics currently available and how these technologies can provide a positive impact on patient care.

Uterine Factors   57

Carolyn R. Jaslow

> Uterine anomalies are one of the most common parental causes of recurrent pregnancy loss, occurring in about 19% of patients. Congenital

uterine anomalies are most likely caused by HOX gene mutations, although the mechanism is probably polygenic. There are no known environmental causes other than estrogenic endocrine disruptors such as diethylstilbestrol. Acquired uterine anomalies may result from uterine trauma (adhesions) or benign growths of the myometrium (fibroids) or endometrium (polyps). Although randomized controlled trials are lacking, surgical treatment is recommended for repair of uterine septa, and for removal of severe adhesions and submucosal fibroids, especially if no other causes are identified.

Mid-Trimester Pregnancy Loss   87

Kelly M. McNamee, Feroza Dawood, and Roy G. Farquharson

Mid-trimester pregnancy loss (MTL) occurs between 12 and 24 weeks' gestation. The true incidence of this pregnancy complication is unknown, because research into MTL in isolation is scarce, although the estimated incidence has been noted to be 2% to 3% of pregnancies. A comprehensive preconceptual screening protocol is recommended, because the cause for an MTL may be present in isolation or combined (dual pathology), and is often heterogeneous. Patients with a history of MTL are at an increased risk of future miscarriage and preterm delivery. This risk is increased further depending on the number of associative factors diagnosed.

Endocrine Basis for Recurrent Pregnancy Loss   103

Raymond W. Ke

Common endocrinopathies are a frequent contributor to spontaneous and recurrent miscarriage. Although the diagnostic criteria for luteal phase defect (LPD) is still controversial, treatment of patients with both recurrent pregnancy loss and LPD using progestogen in early pregnancy seems beneficial. For patients who are hypothyroid, thyroid hormone replacement therapy along with careful monitoring in the preconceptual and early pregnancy period is associated with improved outcome. Women with polycystic ovary syndrome (PCOS) have an increased risk of pregnancy loss. Management of PCOS with normalization of weight or metformin seems to reduce the risk of pregnancy loss.

Antiphospholipid Antibody Syndrome   113

William H. Kutteh and Candace D. Hinote

Antiphospholipid antibodies (aPLs) are acquired antibodies directed against negatively charged phospholipids. Obstetric antiphospholipid antibody syndrome (APS) is diagnosed in the presence of certain clinical features in conjunction with positive laboratory findings. Obstetric APS is one of the most commonly identified causes of recurrent pregnancy loss. Thus, obstetric APS is distinguished from APS in other organ systems where the most common manifestation is thrombosis. Several pathophysiologic mechanisms of action of aPLs have been described. This article discusses the diagnostic and obstetric challenges of obstetric APS, proposed pathophysiologic mechanisms of APS during pregnancy, and the management of women during and after pregnancy.

Inherited Thrombophilias and Adverse Pregnancy Outcomes: A Review of Screening Patterns and Recommendations 133

William B. Davenport and William H. Kutteh

> Historically, much controversy has existed regarding the association of inherited thrombophilias with adverse pregnancy outcomes. The current guidelines do not recommend screening unless a personal history of venous thromboembolism is present, but the authors' survey of physician screening patterns has suggested that up to 40% of physicians may screen contrary to the current guidelines. This article summarizes the existing evidence for each inherited thrombophilia and reviews the current guidelines.

Recurrent Miscarriage Clinics 145

M.M.J. Van den Berg, Rosa Vissenberg, and Mariëtte Goddijn

> A recurrent miscarriage clinic offers specialist investigation and treatment of women with recurrent first- and second-trimester miscarriages. Consultant-led clinics provide a dedicated and focused service to couples who have experienced at least two prior miscarriages. The best treatment strategy for couples with recurrent miscarriage is to discuss a treatment plan for a future pregnancy. Evidence-based up-to-date guidelines are required to reduce ineffective management of recurrent miscarriage couples, including overdiagnostics and underdiagnostics. Scientific research is necessary to study the effectiveness of new interventions, to study patient preferences, and to evaluate health care and costs or other outcomes.

Unexplained Recurrent Pregnancy Loss 157

Sotirios H. Saravelos and Lesley Regan

> Women with unexplained recurrent pregnancy loss (RPL) represent a highly heterogeneous group of patients. Past studies have investigated systemic endocrine and immunologic mechanisms as potential causes for pregnancy loss in unexplained RPL, while exciting new work has focused on spermatozoal, embryonic, and endometrial characteristics to explain the regulation of implantation and subsequent pregnancy loss. In the clinical and research context, stratification of women with unexplained RPL according to whether they have a high probability of pathologic status will help select women who are most appropriate for further investigation and potential future treatment.

Index 167

OBSTETRICS AND GYNECOLOGY CLINICS

FORTHCOMING ISSUES

June 2014
Addiction Disorders in Pregnancy
William Rayburn and Hillary Connery,
Editors

September 2014
Gynecologic Pelvic Pain
Mary McLennan, *Editor*

December 2014
Infectious Diseases in Pregnancy
Geeta Swamy, *Editor*

RECENT ISSUES

December 2013
Procedures in the Office Setting
Tony Ogburn and Besty Taylor, *Editors*

September 2013
Breast Disorders
Victoria L. Green and Patrice M. Weiss,
Editors

June 2013
**HPV, Colposcopy, and Prevention of
Squamous Anogenital Tract Malignancy**
Alan G. Waxman and Maria Lina Diaz,
Editors

Foreword

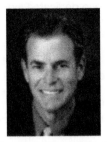

William F. Rayburn, MD, MBA
Consulting Editor

This unique issue of the *Obstetrics and Gynecology Clinics of North America*, guest edited by Dr. William Kutteh, deals with an update on the evaluation and treatment for recurrent pregnancy loss. Recurrent pregnancy loss typically is defined as two or more consecutive pregnancy losses and occurs in approximately 1% of women attempting to bear a child. Recurrent early pregnancy loss is often heterogeneous in origin and is frustrating for the couple, the patients, and clinicians.

For patients with recurrent pregnancy loss, it is reasonable to offer a basic evaluation. As reviewed nicely in this text, the evaluation of women with recurrent pregnancy loss should consider the following factors: antiphospholipid syndrome, endocrine or metabolic imbalances, exposure to toxins and drugs, genetic abnormalities, immunologic disorders, pelvic infections, thrombophilia, and uterine abnormalities. Laboratory studies should include testing for lupus anticoagulant, anticardiolipin antibodies, and microarray genetic testing. Those couples affected by chromosomal abnormalities should be counseled about the risk of recurring abortion and offered prenatal genetic studies as well as considered for newer assisted reproductive technologies for future pregnancies. Cultures for bacteria or viruses and tests for glucose intolerance, antibodies to infectious agents, antinuclear antibodies, antithyroid antibodies, paternal human leukocyte antigen status, or maternal antipaternal antibodies are generally not beneficial.

The authors describe how corrective surgery for uterine defects or a presumed incompetent cervix may be reasonable when such defects appear to interfere with implantation, pregnancy growth, or pregnancy retention. The role of luteal phase defect is controversial, and supplementation with progesterone is of unproven efficacy. Immunoglobulin and paternal leukocyte therapies are not effective in preventing recurrent pregnancy loss.

Nearly half of couples who complete this evaluation will not have an identifiable cause. Informative and supportive counseling appears to play an important role and may lead to the best pregnancy outcomes. Couples with unexplained recurrent pregnancy loss should be counseled regarding the potential for successful pregnancy without treatment. The risk of recurrent abortion after two successive losses remains stable with future pregnancies.

Obstet Gynecol Clin N Am 41 (2014) ix–x
http://dx.doi.org/10.1016/j.ogc.2013.11.001
obgyn.theclinics.com

Contributors to this issue represent some of the field's most dedicated clinicians and investigators, most of whom have spent their entire careers working with couples affected by repeated losses. I am grateful to Dr. Kutteh and these dedicated individuals for their willingness to contribute to this special issue.

William F. Rayburn, MD, MBA
Professor and Chair
Department of Obstetrics and Gynecology
Associate Dean
Continuing Medical Education and Professional Development
University of New Mexico School of Medicine
MSC10 5580, 1 University of New Mexico
Albuquerque, NM 87131-0001, USA

E-mail address:
wrayburn@salud.unm.edu

Preface

Recurrent Pregnancy Loss

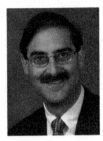

William H. Kutteh, MD, PhD, HCLD
Editor

This issue of the *Obstetrics and Gynecology Clinics of North America* focuses on the advances in the evaluation and management of recurrent pregnancy loss (RPL) that have emerged within the last few years. Although spontaneous pregnancy loss occurs in approximately 15% to 20% of clinically recognized pregnancies in reproductive-aged women, RPL occurs in 2% to 5% of the same population.[1] Recent reports on large populations of women with RPL have helped to characterize the incidence and diversity of this heterogeneous disorder, and a definite cause of pregnancy loss can be established on over 50% of all couples after a thorough evaluation.[2] New diagnostic strategies, which include 23-chromosome microarray genetic testing of the products of conception in failed pregnancies, offer the promise of understanding the cause of most pregnancy losses.[3] These recent advances, combined with the contributions from the authors in this issue of the *Obstetrics and Gynecology Clinics of North America* and many others interested in this field, led to the release of the long-awaited publication on evaluation and treatment of RPL from the Practice Committee of the American Society for Reproductive Medicine.[4] A complete evaluation will include investigations into genetic, anatomic, immunologic, endocrinologic, and iatrogenic factors. The occurrence of RPL may induce significant emotional distress and clinicians must be diligent in making intensive supportive care available in some cases. With a directed approach to diagnosis and careful treatment, a successful outcome will occur in more than two-thirds of all couples.[5]

Miscarriages are considered any loss before 20 weeks (North America) or 24 weeks (Europe) of gestation. Embryonic losses are those that occur before 10 gestational weeks, and fetal losses occur from 10 to 20 (or 24) gestational weeks. Later pregnancy losses are considered stillbirths and will not be a topic covered in this issue. Prior pregnancy history is an important prognostic factor: primary RPL is diagnosed in those couples who have never had a previous viable infant, whereas those couples with secondary RPL have previously delivered a pregnancy beyond 20 gestational weeks and

Obstet Gynecol Clin N Am 41 (2014) xi–xiii
http://dx.doi.org/10.1016/j.ogc.2013.10.009
0889-8545/14/$ – see front matter © 2014 Published by Elsevier Inc.

then suffered subsequent losses. Tertiary RPL is used to identify those couples with multiple miscarriages interspersed with normal pregnancies.

The contributors to this issue represent some of the world's most dedicated clinicians and investigators. Most of them have spent their entire careers working with couples affected by RPL. Ole Christiansen, an obstetrician gynecologist who manages patients with miscarriage through the busy Fertility Clinic Rigshospitalet in Copenhagen, has contributed an article on methods and flaws of RPL research. Roy Farquharson, consultant gynecologist, serves on the National Institute for Health and Clinical Excellence and sees patients at the Liverpool Women's Hospital's Miscarriage Clinic. His group has contributed a chapter on mid trimester pregnancy loss. Mariëtte Goddijn, a reproductive gynecologist at Amsterdam Medical Center Recurrent Miscarriage Program and coordinator of the ESHRE Special Interest Group for Early Pregnancy, has contributed an article on establishing a recurrent miscarriage program. Lesley Regan, Clinical Professor at the Imperial College in London has contributed a chapter on dealing with couples that are diagnosed with unexplained recurrent miscarriage.

A number of investigators and collaborators with the Center for the Study of Recurrent Pregnancy Loss in Memphis, TN have made valuable contributions to this publication. Carolyn Jaslow, an active teacher and research professor of Reproductive Biology at Rhodes College, has made significant contributions in characterizing the causes of RPL and has added a review on anatomic causes of RPL. Brett Davenport has taken his data and provided a contemporary review of thrombophilias and their potential role in RPL. Raymond Ke, a true reproductive endocrinologist and practitioner in our RPL Center in Memphis, has written a concise update on hormonal factors and RPL. Paul Brezina, director of the reproductive genetics program at our RPL Center in Memphis, has provided a review of genetic trends in our field that will impact patient care in reproductive medicine. To summarize current research, we have devoted a summary chapter to the latest strategies for the management of early pregnancy loss.

Finally, many thanks to William Rayburn for the opportunity to guest edit this issue on Recurrent Pregnancy Loss for *Obstetrics and Gynecology Clinics of North America*. It has been a pleasure working with him and the staff at Elsevier to make this issue a reality. On behalf of all the contributors to this issue, we hope that this update will be informative for you and beneficial for the patients that you care for with RPL.

William H. Kutteh, MD, PhD, HCLD
Vanderbilt University School of Medicine
Recurrent Pregnancy Loss Center
Fertility Associates of Memphis
Memphis, TN, USA

E-mail address:
wkutteh@fertilitymemphis.com

REFERENCES

1. Stephenson MD, Kutteh WH. Evaluation and management of recurrent early pregnancy loss. Clin Obstet Gynecol 2007;50:132–45.
2. Jaslow CR, Carney JL, Kutteh WH. Diagnostic factors identified in 1020 women with two versus three or more recurrent pregnancy losses. Fertil Steril 2010;93: 1234–43.

3. Brezina PR, Kutteh WH. Recurrent early pregnancy loss. In: Flacone T, Hurd WW, editors. Clinical reproductive medicine and surgery: a practical guide. 2nd edition. New York: Springer Science + Business Media; Chapter 13. p. 197–208.
4. The Practice Committee of the American Society for Reproductive Medicine. Evaluation and treatment of recurrent pregnancy loss: a committee opinion. Fertil Steril 2012;98:1103–11.
5. Lund M, Kamper-Jorgensen M, Nielsen HS, et al. Prognosis for live birth in women with recurrent miscarriage: what is the best measure of success? Obstet Gynecol 2012;119:37–43.

Classic and Cutting-Edge Strategies for the Management of Early Pregnancy Loss

Paul R. Brezina, MD, MBA*, William H. Kutteh, MD, PhD, HCLD

KEYWORDS

- Recurrent pregnancy loss • RPL • Miscarriage • Spontaneous abortion • Aneuploid
- Antiphospholipid • Lupus anticoagulant • Heparin

KEY POINTS

- There are few conditions in medicine associated with more heartache to patients than recurrent pregnancy loss (RPL).
- The management of early RPL is a formidable clinical challenge for physicians.
- Great strides have been made in characterizing the incidence and diversity of this heterogeneous disorder, and a definite cause of pregnancy loss can be established in more than half of couples after a thorough evaluation.
- In this review, current data are evaluated and a clear roadmap is provided for the evaluation and treatment of RPL.

INTRODUCTION

Recurrent early pregnancy loss is a profound personal tragedy to couples seeking parenthood and a formidable clinical challenge to their physician. When to evaluate a couple and what constitutes a complete evaluation is, at the time of the writing of this article, in a state of flux. The American College of Obstetricians and Gynecologists (ACOG) has withdrawn its 2001 Practice Bulletin on early RPL and has not issued a replacement for more than 1 year. The American Society for Reproductive Medicine

Disclosure: Contributors: P.R. Brezina primarily searched the literature. P.R. Brezina wrote the first draft of the article; W.H. Kutteh edited the article and advised on the content of the article, assisted in the literature search, and contributed to the writing of the article. P.R. Brezina is guarantor.
Competing Interests: All authors have completed the Unified Competing Interest form and declare: no support from any organization for the submitted work; no financial relationships with any organizations that might have an interest in the submitted work in the previous 3 years; and no other relationships or activities that could appear to have influenced the submitted work.
Sources of Funding: None.
Fertility Associates of Memphis, 80 Humphreys Center, Suite 307, Memphis, TN 38120, USA
* Corresponding author.
E-mail address: pbrezina@fertilitymemphis.com

Obstet Gynecol Clin N Am 41 (2014) 1–18
http://dx.doi.org/10.1016/j.ogc.2013.10.011
0889-8545/14/$ – see front matter © 2014 Elsevier Inc. All rights reserved.

obgyn.theclinics.com

(ASRM) has recently released a committee opinion after extensively evaluating available evidence over a 7-year period.[1]

Although spontaneous abortion occurs in approximately 15% of clinically diagnosed pregnancies of reproductive-aged women, recurrent pregnancy loss (RPL) occurs in about 1% to 2% of this same population.[2] Great strides have been made in characterizing the incidence and diversity of this heterogeneous disorder, and a definite cause of pregnancy loss can be established in more than half of couples after a thorough evaluation.[3,4] A complete evaluation includes investigations into genetic, endocrinologic, anatomic, immunologic, and iatrogenic causes. The occurrence of RPL may induce significant emotional distress, and, in some cases, intensive supportive care may be necessary. Successful outcomes occur in more than two-thirds of all couples.[4,5]

DEFINITION OF PREGNANCY LOSS

The traditional definition of RPL included those couples with 3 or more spontaneous, consecutive pregnancy losses. Ectopic and molar pregnancies are not included. The ASRM has defined RPL as "a distinct disorder defined by 2 or more failed clinical pregnancies."[1] For purposes of determining if an evaluation for RPL is appropriate, pregnancy "is defined as a clinical pregnancy documented by ultrasonography or histopathological examination."[1] Several studies have recently indicated that the risk of recurrent miscarriage after 2 successive losses is similar to the risk of miscarriage in women after 3 successive losses; thus, it is reasonable to start an evaluation after 2 or more consecutive spontaneous miscarriages to determine the cause of their pregnancy loss, especially when the woman is older than 35 years of age, or when the couple have had difficulty conceiving.[6]

Those couples with primary RPL have never had a previous viable infant, whereas those with secondary recurrent loss have previously delivered a pregnancy beyond 20 weeks and then suffered subsequent losses. Tertiary recurrent loss refers to those women who have multiple miscarriages interspersed with normal pregnancies.

RECURRENCE RISK

The main concerns of couples with recurrent miscarriage when they present to our RPL center is to find the cause and to establish the risk of recurrence. In a first pregnancy, the overall risk of loss of a clinically recognized pregnancy loss is 15%.[7,8] However, the true risk of early pregnancy loss is estimated to be around 50% because of the high rate of losses that occur before the first missed menstrual period. Furthermore, as women age, this rate likely increases because of chromosomal errors introduced through meiotic nondisjunction errors during oocyte maturation. Studies that evaluated the frequency of pregnancy loss,[7,8] based on highly sensitive tests for quantitative human chorionic gonadotropin (hCG), indicated that the total clinical and preclinical losses in women aged 20 to 30 years is approximately 25%, whereas the loss rate in women aged 40 years or more is at least double that figure. The ability to predict the risk of recurrence is influenced by several factors, including maternal age, parental and fetal karyotypes, the gestational age at which prior losses occurred, and the presence of various maternal laboratory findings.[8–14]

CAUSES, DIAGNOSIS, AND TREATMENT OF RPL
Introduction

Traditionally, the chief causes of RPL have been believed to be embryonic chromosomal abnormalities, maternal anatomic abnormalities such as a uterine septum, luteal phase defects, and antiphospholipid (aPL) antibodies. Other factors such as infection and a hypercoaguable state have also been considered but to a lesser degree.

When to initiate an RPL workup has been a source of recent debate. Classically, conducting a workup for RPL was recommended after 3 miscarriages. Recent data do not necessarily support this traditional evaluation protocol.[15,16] The evaluation of healthy women after a single loss is usually not recommended, because this a common, sporadic event. However, the risk of another pregnancy loss after 2 miscarriages is only slightly lower (24%–29%) than that of women with 3 or more spontaneous abortions (31%–33%).[7] Therefore, evaluation and treatment can reasonably be started after 2 consecutive miscarriages.[1,4] Furthermore, additional testing such as chromosomal testing of the products of conception from a second miscarriage may confer a cost-savings measure.[15,16] Based on available data, we outline a new strategy for the workup of RPL (Figs. 1 and 2).

An evaluation of a patient with RPL should always include a complete history, including documentation of previous pregnancies, any pathologic tests that were performed on previous miscarriages, any evidence of chronic or acute infections or diseases, any recent physical or emotional trauma, history of cramping or bleeding with a previous miscarriage, any family history of pregnancy loss, and any previous gynecologic surgery or complicating factor. A summary of the diagnosis and management of RPL includes an investigation of genetic, endocrinologic, anatomic, immunologic, and iatrogenic causes (Table 1).

We outline a proposed algorithm for the evaluation and treatment of RPL (see Fig. 1). Under this new schema, no diagnostic/therapeutic action is recommended after 1 miscarriage. Fetal karyotype is recommended to be obtained after either the second consecutive or third nonconsecutive miscarriage. Products of conception (POC)

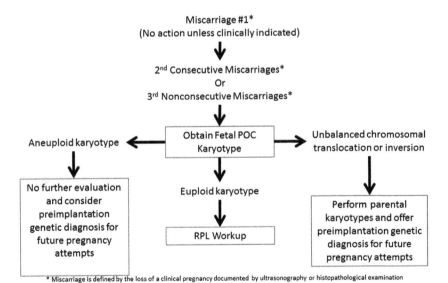

Fig. 1. Initial evaluation for early RPL. An algorithm for the initial evaluation of early RPL. Arrows are provided that guide the reader through various outcomes possible during the RPL evaluation and appropriate next steps in diagnostic management. (*From* Brezina PR, Kutteh WH. Recurrent early pregnancy loss. In: Falcone T, Hurd W, editors. Clinical reproductive medicine and surgery: a practical guide. 2nd edition. New York: Springer; 2013; with permission.)

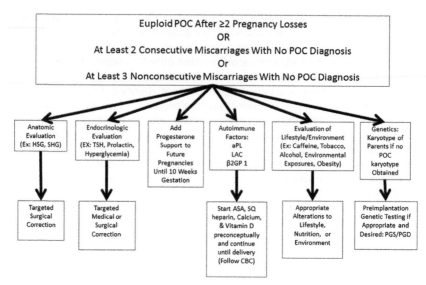

Fig. 2. Workup for early RPL. An algorithm for the full workup of early RPL. Arrows are provided that guide the reader through various outcomes possible during the RPL evaluation and appropriate next steps in diagnostic and therapeutic management. (*From* Brezina PR, Kutteh WH. Recurrent early pregnancy loss. In: Falcone T, Hurd W, editors. Clinical reproductive medicine and surgery: a practical guide. 2nd edition. New York: Springer; 2013; with permission.)

Table 1 Diagnosis and management of RPL		
Cause	**Diagnostic Evaluation**	**Therapy**
Genetic	Karyotype partners Karyotype products of conception	Genetic counseling Donor gametes, preimplantation genetic diagnosis
Anatomic	Hysterosalpingography Hysteroscopy Sonohysterography Transvaginal three-dimensional ultrasonography	Septum transection Myomectomy Lysis of adhesions
Endocrinologic	Midluteal progesterone Thyroid-stimulating hormone Prolactin Hemoglobin A_{1C}	Progesterone Levothyroxine Bromocriptine, dostinex Metformin
Immunologic	Lupus anticoagulant Antiphospholipid antibodies Anti-β_2 glycoprotein	Aspirin Heparin + aspirin
Psychological	Interview	Support groups
Iatrogenic	Tobacco, alcohol use, obesity Exposure to toxins, chemicals	Eliminate consumption Eliminate exposure

to send for karyotype may be obtained from early nonviable pregnancies either via traditional dilation and curettage. POC may be sent for traditional karyotype or, as we recommend, be sent for 23 chromosome pair microarray evaluation.

The results of this POC karyotype guide further evaluation. If the POC are found to be aneuploid, no further evaluation or treatment is recommended at that juncture, because the cause for the loss is known, although all future early miscarriages should also be subject to karyotypic evaluation. If an unbalanced chromosomal translocation or inversion is identified in the fetal POC, then the workup focuses on performing parental karyotypes and offering appropriate therapeutic options, such as preimplantation genetic testing. If the fetal POC are found to be chromosomally normal, then a full RPL workup is to be performed. If the fetal POC karyotypes have not been performed, then we recommend a full RPL workup after at least 2 consecutive miscarriages or at least 3 nonconsecutive miscarriages. The full RPL workup is outlined in **Fig. 2**.

What constitutes a full RPL is a topic of debate. We recommend including an anatomic evaluation, endocrinologic evaluation, testing for autoimmune factors, evaluating lifestyle and environmental factors, and obtaining parental karyotypes if the karyotypic status of previous POC is unknown. Not included in this evaluation are more controversial types of testing and therapies such as those dealing with microbiological factors, thrombophilic factors, immunotherapy, and other evaluations, although these may be appropriate in certain clinical situations. In the following sections, the physiologic background, diagnostic approaches, and therapy for the various components of our proposed RPL workup are described. In addition, other more controversial proposed causes of RPL are addressed (**Box 1**).

ANATOMIC CAUSES OF RPL

Anatomic causes of RPL are typically diagnosed using hysterosalpingography (HSG) or sonohysterography. Hysteroscopy, laparoscopy, or magnetic resonance imaging can supplement these tests as needed. Recently, transvaginal three-dimensional ultrasonography has been introduced and has allowed an accurate and noninvasive diagnosis of congenital uterine anomalies. The treatment of congenital and acquired uterine anomalies often involves corrective surgery (**Box 2**).

Congenital Malformations

Congenital malformations of the reproductive tract result from failure to complete bilateral duct elongation, fusion, canalization, or septal resorption of the müllerian

---

Box 1
Pearls

1. A complete evaluation for RPL shows possible causes in 60% of cases.

2. The complete evaluation (genetic, endocrinologic, anatomic, immunologic, and iatrogenic) should be initiated when the decision to evaluate a couple is made.

3. Couples with primary RPL have identifiable causes just as frequently as couples with secondary RPL; therefore, all couples should be evaluated.

4. Women with 2 losses have identifiable problems just as frequently as women with 3 or more losses; thus, evaluation for causes may be initiated after 2 losses.

5. If no cause is identified after a complete evaluation, 65% of couples have a successful subsequent pregnancy.

Box 2
Anatomic causes of RPL

1. Congenital malformations of the reproductive tract
2. Intrauterine adhesions
3. Intrauterine masses, including fibroids or polyps
4. Incompetent cervix

---

ducts. Müllerian anomalies were found in 8% to 10% of women who had had 3 or more consecutive spontaneous abortions who underwent HSG or hysteroscopic examination of their uteri.[3,4,17] Inadequate vascularity compromising the developing placenta and reduced intraluminal volume have been theorized as possible mechanisms leading to pregnancy loss.

The most common congenital abnormality associated with pregnancy loss is the septate uterus.[18] The spontaneous abortion rate is high, averaging about 65% of pregnancies in some studies.[19] A septum is primarily composed of fibromuscular tissue, which is poorly vascularized. This lack of vascularization may compromise decidual and placental growth. Alternatively, a uterine septum may impair fetal growth as a result of reduced endometrial capacity or a distorted endometrial cavity.[19] Uncontrolled studies suggest that resection of the uterine septum results in higher delivery rates than in women without treatment. Other congenital abnormalities, such as uterine didelphys and bicornuate and unicornuate uterus, are more frequently associated with later trimester losses or preterm delivery.

Intrauterine Adhesions

Intrauterine trauma resulting from endometrial curettage or endometritis is associated with a risk for the development of adhesions. Intrauterine adhesions (synechiae) are an acquired uterine defect, which has been associated with recurrent miscarriage. The severity of adhesions may range form minimal to complete ablation of the endometrial cavity. The term Asherman syndrome is often used to describe intrauterine adhesions associated with oligomenorrhea or amenorrhea. These adhesions are believed to interfere with the normal placentation and are treated with hysteroscopic resection. The insertion of an intrauterine balloon catheter for 1 week is recommended by some physicians after resection of synechiae to help prevent reformation of adhesions. During this time, antibiotic prophylaxis with doxycycline (100 mg twice a day) is given to prevent endometritis. Patients may also be given estrogen and progestin for 1 month.

Intrauterine Masses

Intrauterine cavity abnormalities, such as submucosal leiomyomas and polyps, can contribute to pregnancy loss. Depending on the leiomyoma size and location, it may partially obliterate or alter the contour of the intrauterine cavity, providing a poorly vascularized endometrium for implantation or otherwise compromising placental development. Uterine leiomyomas and polyps may also act like an intrauterine device, causing subacute endometritis. Until recently, it was believed that only submucous leiomyomas should be surgically removed before subsequent attempts at pregnancy. However, several recent studies investigating the implantation rate in women undergoing in vitro fertilization (IVF) have clearly shown decreased implantation, with intramural leiomyomas in the range of 30 mm.[20] When smaller leiomyomas are identified, it is unclear if myomectomy is beneficial.[21]

Incompetence Cervix

Cervical incompetence can be considered as an acquired uterine anomaly that is associated with RPL. The diagnosis of cervical incompetence is based on the presence of painless cervical dilation, resulting in the inability of the uterine cervix to retain a pregnancy. Cervical incompetence commonly causes pregnancy loss in the second, rather than first, trimester. It may be associated with congenital uterine abnormalities, such as septate or bicornuate uterus. It is postulated that most cases occur as a result of surgical trauma to the cervix from conization, loop electrosurgical excision procedures, overdilation of the cervix during pregnancy termination, or obstetric lacerations.[22]

ENDOCRINOLOGIC CAUSES OF RPL

Endocrine factors may contribute to 8% to 12% of RPL. Therefore, an endocrinologic evaluation is a critical component of the RPL workup (**Box 3**).

Luteal Phase Deficiency

Maintenance of early pregnancy depends on the production of progesterone by the corpus luteum. Between 7 and 9 weeks of gestation, the developing placenta takes over the progesterone production. Luteal phase deficiency (LPD) is defined as an inability of the corpus luteum to secrete progesterone in high enough amounts or for too short a duration. The preponderance of evidence suggests that LPD is a preovulatory event most likely linked to an alteration in the preovulatory estrogen stimulation, which may indicate poor oocyte quality and a poorly functioning corpus luteum.[23,24] Classically, the diagnosis is based on results of endometrial biopsy, although this is not recommended as a diagnostic modality. Most investigators advocate the measurement of serum progesterone levels in the luteal phase for the diagnosis of LPD, with levels lower than 10 ng/mL considered abnormal.[25] However, progesterone levels are subject to large fluctuations because of pulsatile release of the luteinizing hormone (LH). Moreover, there is a lack of correlation between serum levels of progesterone and endometrial histology.[26] Although conflicting data exist, a recent Cochrane review evaluating 15 trials concluded that there was a benefit to the routine administration of progesterone to all women with a history of RPL.[27,28] Progesterone is available either as intravaginal suppositories (50–100 mg twice daily starting the third day after LH surge and continuing for 8–10 weeks) or as intramuscular (IM) injections (50 mg IM daily).

Box 3
Endocrinologic causes of RPL

1. Luteal phase deficiency

2. Untreated hypothyroidism

3. Abnormal glucose metabolism

4. Hyperprolactinemia

5. Diminished ovarian reserve

Untreated Hypothyroidism

Untreated hypothyroidism may increase the risk of miscarriage. A study of more than 700 patients with RPL identified 7.6% with hypothyroidism.[29] Hypothyroidism is easily diagnosed with a sensitive thyroid-stimulating hormone (TSH) test, and patients should be treated to become euthyroid (defined for the purposes of RPL as between 1.0 and 2.5 uIU/mL) before attempting a next pregnancy.[1,30] It has also been suggested that thyroid antibodies are increased in women with RPL. A retrospective study of 700 patients with RPL[31] showed that 158 women had antithyroid antibodies but only 23 of those women had clinical hypothyroidism from an abnormal TSH value. The presence of antithyroid antibodies may imply abnormal T-cell function, and therefore, more of an immune dysfunction rather than an endocrine disorder may be responsible for the pregnancy losses. The Endocrine Society recommends that patients with RPL be treated to keep a TSH level of between 1.0 and 2.5 uIU/mL in the first trimester.[30] For TSH levels found to be between 2.5 and 10 mIU/mL, a starting levothyroxine dose of at least 50 μg/d is recommended.[30]

Abnormal Glucose Metabolism

Patients with poorly controlled diabetes are known to have an increased risk of spontaneous miscarriage, which is reduced to normal spontaneous loss rates when women are euglycemic preconceptually.[32] Testing for fasting insulin and glucose is simple, and treatment with insulin-sensitizing agents can reduce the risk of recurrent miscarriage.[33] More recently, determining the average load of blood glucose through testing of hemoglobin A_{1C} has become an increasingly used modality to evaluate insulin resistance.[1] Because there is strong evidence that obesity or insulin resistance is associated with an increased risk of miscarriage, weight reduction in obese women is a first step in the treatment. Metformin seems to improve pregnancy outcome, but the evidence for this treatment is limited to a few cohort studies. Metformin is a category B medication in the first trimester of pregnancy and seems to be safe. Other endocrine abnormalities, such as thyroid disorders and diabetes, should be corrected before conception.

Hyperprolactinemia

Normal circulating levels of prolactin may play an important role in maintaining early pregnancy. Data from animal studies suggest that increased prolactin levels may adversely affect corpus luteal function; however, this concept has not been proved in humans.[34] A recent study of 64 hyperprolactinemic women showed that bromocriptine therapy was associated with a higher rate of successful pregnancy and that prolactin levels were significantly higher in women who miscarried.[35]

Diminished Ovarian Reserve

Follicle stimulating hormone (FSH) is believed to be a marker of the number of follicles available for recruitment on any given menstrual cycle. Therefore, increased levels of FSH in the early follicular phase of the menstrual cycle are representative of diminished ovarian reserve; a condition in which a low number of follicular units are available for recruitment. More recently, other markers, such as decreased anti-müllerian hormone, have been introduced to identify diminished ovarian reserve. Although the frequency of increased day 3 FSH levels in women with recurrent miscarriage is similar to the frequency in the infertile population, the prognosis of recurrent miscarriages is worsened with increased day 3 FSH levels.[36] Although no treatment is available, testing may be helpful in women older than 35 years with RPL, and appropriate counseling should follow.

AUTOIMMUNE/THROMBOTIC FACTORS AS THE CAUSE OF RPL
Immunologic Disorders

Autoimmune factors: maternal response to self
In some instances, there is a failure in normal control mechanisms that prevent an immune reaction against self, resulting in an autoimmune response (**Box 4**).[37] Autoantibodies to phospholipids, thyroid antigens, nuclear antigens, and others have been investigated as possible causes for pregnancy loss.[29] aPL antibodies include the lupus anticoagulant, anti-β_2 glycoprotein I antibodies, and anticardiolipin antibodies. There is still controversy concerning testing for other phospholipids, but an increasing number of studies suggest that antibodies to phosphatidyl serine are also associated with pregnancy loss.[38] Women with systemic lupus erythematosus and aPL antibodies have increased risks for miscarriage compared with those with lupus and negative aPL antibodies.[39]

Antiphospholipid Antibody Syndrome

Antiphospholipid antibody syndrome (APS) is an autoimmune condition characterized by the production of moderate to high levels of aPL antibodies and certain clinical features (**Table 2**).[40] The presence of aPL antibodies (anticardiolipin and lupus anticoagulant) during pregnancy is a major risk factor for adverse pregnancy outcome.[41] In a large meta-analysis of studies of couples with recurrent abortion, the incidence of APS was between 15% and 20% compared with about 5% in nonpregnant women without a history of obstetric complications.[42,43]

Several mechanisms have been proposed by which aPL antibodies might mediate pregnancy loss. Classically, it was believed that aPL antibodies induced thromboses in vessels surrounding the placental-maternal unit, resulting in placental infarction and fetal death. However, recent data have suggested that the primary mechanism by which aPL antibodies lead to miscarriage may be via a deleterious effect conferred directly on trophoblastic cells or endothelial cells.[44,45] aPL antibodies can interact with cultured human vascular endothelial cells with resultant injury or activation.[44] Furthermore, aPL antibodies have been shown to inhibit secretion of human placental chorionic gonadotropin and to inhibit the expression of trophoblast cell adhesion molecules (α_1 and α_5 integrins, E and VE cadherins).[45] These mechanisms could explain RPL secondary to aPL antibodies early in the first trimester.[42,46,47]

APS is treated with a combination of low-dose heparin (5000–10,000 units subcutaneously every 12 hours), and low-dose aspirin (81 mg by mouth daily) seems to be effective and may reduce pregnancy loss by 54% in women with APS.[42,46,47] Aspirin alone does not seem to reduce miscarriage rates.[48] Unfractionated heparin is preferred to low-molecular-weight heparin, based on available data.[49]

Box 4
Autoimmune factors as the cause of RPL

1. Antiphospholipid antibody syndrome
   a. Anticardiolipin antibodies
   b. Lupus anticoagulant
   c. β_2 Glycoprotein antibodies

Table 2
Clinical and laboratory characteristics of antiphospholipid antibody syndrome

Clinical	Laboratory
Pregnancy morbidity	IgG anticardiolipin[a]
≥1 unexplained death at ≥10 wk or	IgM anticardiolipin[a]
Delivery at ≤34 wk with severe pregnancy-induced hypertension or	Positive lupus anticoagulant test
≥3 losses before 10 wk	IgG anti-β_2 glycoprotein 1[a]
Thrombosis	IgM anti-β_2 glycoprotein 1[a]
Venous	—
Arterial, including stroke	—

Patients should have at least 1 clinical and 1 laboratory feature at some time in the course of their disease. Laboratory tests should be positive on at least 2 occasions.
  [a] ≥99th percentile.
  Modified from Miyakis S, Lockshin MD, Atsumi T, et al. International consensus statement on an update of the classification criteria for definite antiphospholipid syndrome (APS). J Thromb Haemost 2006;4:295–306; with permission.

Treatment with steroids is not recommended based on current evidence.[42,50] Aspirin should be started preconceptually, and heparin should be started after the first positive pregnancy test.[46] Treatment should be continued until the time of delivery, because these women are at an increased risk for thrombosis. Postpartum thrombo-prophylaxis is reasonable for a short interval to prevent thrombosis when the risk is high.[43] The adverse reactions associated with heparin include bleeding, thrombocytopenia, and osteoporosis with fracture. Calcium (600 mg twice daily) with added vitamin D supplementation (400 IU daily) and weight-bearing exercise are encouraged to decrease the risk of osteoporosis. In any pregnant woman starting on heparin, the platelet count should be monitored weekly for the first 2 weeks after initiation, and after any dosage change. Women with APS should consider avoiding the use of estrogen-containing oral contraceptives in the future.[51]

Immunotherapy

Immunotherapy for alloimmune disorders is based on the hypothesis that spontaneous abortion occurs because of a failure of maternal immunologic adaptation to the developing conceptus, resulting in a form of transplantation rejection. Although some randomized double-blind studies have shown an increase with therapies such as paternal leukocyte immunization, trophoblast immune infusion, intravenous intralipid therapy, and immunoglobulin infusion in successful pregnancy outcomes, other have not confirmed these results.[51–53] A Cochrane review of 19 trials of various forms of immunotherapy[54] did not show significant differences between treatment and control groups. There is insufficient evidence to recommend the use of these therapies for RPL. Testing for T_H1 and T_H2 profiles, parental HLA profiles, alloantibodies, natural killer cells, antiparental cytotoxic antibodies, or embryotoxic factor assessment are not clinically justified.

Antinuclear Antibodies

Approximately 10% to 15% of all women have detectable antinuclear antibodies, regardless of their history of pregnancy loss. Their chance of successful pregnancy outcome is not dependent on the presence or absence of antinuclear antibodies.

Treatments such as steroids have been shown to increase the maternal and fetal complications without benefiting live births.[55] Thus, routine testing and treatment of antinuclear antibodies are not indicated.

Microbiological

Certain infectious agents have been identified more frequently in cultures from women who have had spontaneous pregnancy losses.[56] These agents include *Ureaplasma urealyticum*, *Mycoplasma hominis*, and *Chlamydia*. Other less frequent pathogens include *Toxoplasma gondii*, rubella, herpes simplex virus, measles, cytomegalovirus, coxsackievirus, and *Listeria monocytogenes*. None of these pathogens has been causally linked to RPL. Because of the association with sporadic pregnancy losses and the ease of diagnosis, some clinicians test women with RPL and treat for the appropriate pathogen in both parents.

Appropriate antibiotic therapy should be instituted in both parents when cervical infections are identified. Infections with *Mycoplasma*, *Ureaplasma*, and *Chlamydia* are treated with doxycycline, 100 mg twice daily by mouth for 14 days. For those who fail treatment based on a test of cure culture, the options are to extend treatment of both partners to 30 days or to use ofloxacin 300 mg daily for 14 days for both partners.

Thrombotic Disorders

Thrombophilias are believed to be responsible for more than half of maternal venous thromboembolisms in pregnancy; however, ACOG recommends that only patients with a personal or family history of thromboembolic events should be tested.[57]

The recommended evaluations are:

a. Factor V Leiden screening with activated protein C (APC) resistance using a second-generation coagulation assay is probably the most cost-effective approach. Patients with a low APC resistance ratio (<2.0) should then be genotyped for the factor V Leiden mutation
b. Prothrombin G20210A gene mutation using polymerase chain reaction
c. Antithrombin activity with normal levels between 75% and 130%
d. Protein S activity with normal levels between 60% and 145%
e. Protein C activity with normal levels between 75% and 150%

GENETIC FACTORS AS THE CAUSE OF RPL

There are a variety of genetic factors that may result in failure of a pregnancy to develop. These factors include aneuploidy (the gain or loss of a chromosome), chromosomal imbalances as a result of parentally harbored translocations or inversions, deletions or duplications of genetic information within chromosomes, and single-gene mutations. Broadly, genetic factors may be divided into embryonic errors derived from known parental chromosomal abnormalities and embryonic errors that arise de novo in apparently chromosomally normal parents.

Parental Chromosomal Disorders

Parental chromosome anomalies occur in 3% to 5% of couples with RPL as opposed to 0.7% in the general population. These anomalies include translocations, inversions, and the rare ring chromosomes. Balanced translocations are the most common chromosomal abnormalities contributing to RPL.[58] Chromosomal abnormality in 1 of the parents can be found in up to 3% to 5% of couples who experience multiple spontaneous abortions. If no fetal POC are available and the couple have a history of at least 2 consecutive or 3 nonconsecutive fetal losses, we recommend obtaining parental karyotypes. Treatment of parental balanced chromosomal translocations/inversions may be addressed through preimplantation genetic testing, which is addressed later in this article.

Recurrent Aneuploidy

The first chromosomally abnormal abortus was documented in 1961, and since then, a large body of data on the chromosomal status of spontaneous abortuses has accumulated. The overall frequency of chromosome abnormalities in spontaneous abortions is at least 50%.[14,59–62]

Developmental Errors in Euploid Embryos

Another cause of first-trimester miscarriage seems to be failure of chromosomally normal embryos to develop properly. Much as women with müllerian agenesis are chromosomally normal but have a separate developmental abnormality, serious developmental abnormalities that involve vital structures may result in euploid embryos. Small studies have suggested that the rates of significant anatomic abnormalities in chromosomally normal embryos taken from first-trimester miscarriages in women with RPL may exceed 25%.[63]

Preimplantation Genetic Testing

Genetic causes of RPL may be subdivided into embryo abnormalities that are the result of known parental abnormalities (such as parental balanced translocations or inversions) and embryo aneuploidy in parents believed to be chromosomally normal. Preimplantation genetic testing is a technology that is designed to minimize the effects of these and other embryonic genetic abnormalities. Preimplantation genetic testing is accomplished by performing an IVF cycle, removing a cell(s) from the resultant embryos or oocytes, evaluating this cell for genetic abnormalities, and using the results to determine which embryos are ideal for uterine transfer. When a known parental genetic abnormality is identified, as in parental balanced translocations, this practice is referred to as preimplantation genetic diagnosis (PGD). When this process is executed to determine which embryos are aneuploid in parents believed to be chromosomally normal, the procedure is referred to as preimplantation genetic screening (PGS).

PGD for structural aberrations such as translocations and inversions is a generally accepted use of preimplantation genetic testing. In contrast, PGS is more controversial. A 2007 publication in the *New England Journal of Medicine* by Mastenbroek and colleagues[64] showed no benefit to PGS. This study was followed by major medical societies discouraging the routine use of PGS.[65] Since this time, newer technologies, such as microarrays, have been introduced, which are capable of evaluating the ploidy status of all 23 pairs of chromosomes instead of the 9 to 14 pairs of chromosomes evaluated with older fluorescence in situ hybridization technologies.[66] In addition, performing embryo biopsy at the blastocyst, as opposed to the cleavage, stage seems to confer superior pregnancy rates.[67,68] Although recent data evaluating pregnancy rates in RPL patients using 23 chromosome microarrays are encouraging, the routine use of this technology remains controversial.[69,70]

LIFESTYLE ISSUES AND ENVIRONMENTAL TOXINS

Couples experiencing RPL are often concerned that those toxins within the environment may have contributed to their reproductive difficulty. It is important that health care providers, counseling patients about exposures to substances in the environment, have current and accurate information in order to respond to these concerns.

Cigarette Smoking

Cigarette smoking reduces fertility and increases the rate of spontaneous abortion. The data evaluating smoking and miscarriage are extensive and involve approximately 100,000 individuals. The studies suggest a clinically significant detrimental effect of cigarette smoking, which is dose dependent, with a relative risk for miscarriage among moderate smokers (10–20 cigarettes a day) being 1.1 to 1.3.[71] Patients should be aggressively counseled to stop cigarette smoking before attempting pregnancy.

Alcohol Consumption

Alcohol consumption is associated with a risk of spontaneous abortion.[72] The minimum threshold dose for significantly increasing the risk of first-trimester miscarriage seems to be 2 or more alcoholic drinks per week.[73,74] When personal habits, cigarette smoking, and alcohol are used in the same individual, the risk of pregnancy loss may increase 4-fold. Couples should be counseled concerning these habits and strongly encouraged to discontinue these before attempting subsequent conception.[75]

Obesity

Obesity, defined as a body mass index (BMI, calculated as weight in kilograms divided by the square of height in meters) greater than 30, has been associated with an increased risk of miscarriage. Obesity (BMI>30 kg/m^2) has been shown to be an independent risk factor for first-trimester miscarriage.[24] The association is strongest in women with BMI greater than 40. The cause of this phenomenon is unclear. However, many studies have linked obesity to a generalized increase in systemic inflammatory responses.[76]

Caffeine Intake

Several studies have shown that caffeine in excess of 300 mg/d (>2 cups of coffee per day) is associated with a modest increase in spontaneous abortion, but it is not clear if this relationship is causal.[77]

Ionizing Radiation

The studies of atomic bomb survivors in Japan showed that in utero exposure to high-dose radiation increased the risk of spontaneous abortions, premature deliveries, and stillbirths.[78] Diagnostic radiographs in the first trimester delivering less than 5 rad are not teratogenic.[79,80] However, large doses (360–500 rad), used in therapeutic radiation, induce abortion in offspring exposed in utero in most cases. Adverse effects of chronic low-dose radiation on reproduction have not been identified in humans.[80]

OUTCOME

The treatment of RPL should be directed at the cause. Given the good outcome for most couples with unexplained recurrent abortion in the absence of treatment, it is difficult to recommend unproven therapies, especially if they are invasive and expensive. Explanation and appropriate emotional support are possibly the 2 most important aspects of therapy. In 1 study,[17] antenatal counseling and psychological support for couples with recurrent abortion and no abnormal findings resulted in a pregnancy success rate of 86% compared with a success rate of 33% for women who were given no specific antenatal care.

In approximately 60% of all cases of RPL, a complete evaluation shows a possible cause.[3,4] Abnormal findings during the evaluation should be corrected before attempting any subsequent pregnancy. If no cause can be found, most couples have a successful pregnancy outcome with supportive therapy alone.[73] Once a pregnancy occurs, the patient should be monitored closely, with evaluation of quantitative hCG levels at least twice and documentation of adequate progesterone levels. Early sonography should be scheduled, and any encouraging results should be communicated to the couple. In women with a history of RPL, the presence of a normal embryonic heart rate between 6 and 8 gestational weeks that is confirmed with repeat sonography in 1 week is associated with a live birth rate of 82%.[81,82]

Couples who have experienced RPL want to know what caused the miscarriage. Unexplained reproductive failure can lead to anger, guilt, and depression. Anger may be directed toward their physician for not being able to solve their reproductive problems. Feelings of grief and guilt after an early loss are often as intense as those after a stillbirth, and parents experience a grief reaction similar to those associated with the death of an adult. The couple should be assured that exercise, intercourse, and dietary indiscretions do not cause miscarriage. Any questions or concerns that the couple may have about personal habits should be discussed.

The prognosis for women with RPL to deliver with medical therapy is good. A recent study[5] evaluating 987 women with RPL found that the chances of achieving a live birth within 5 years of initial physician consultation was in excess of 80% for women younger than 30 years and approximately 60% to 70% for women aged 31 to 40 years.

Women who suffer RPL have already begun to prepare for their baby, both emotionally and physically, compared with couples with infertility who have never conceived. When a miscarriage occurs, a couple may have great difficulty informing friends or family about the loss. Feelings of hopelessness may continue long after the loss. Patients may continue to grieve and have episodes of depression on the expected due date or the date of the pregnancy loss. Participation in support groups or referral for grief counseling may be beneficial in many cases (SHARE, Pregnancy and Infant Loss Support, http://www.nationalshare.com/).

ACKNOWLEDGMENTS

We thank Drs Raymond Ke and Jianchi Ding for their help with the writing of this article.

REFERENCES

1. The Practice Committee of the American Society for Reproductive Medicine. Evaluation and treatment of recurrent pregnancy loss: a committee opinion. Fertil Steril 2012;98(5):1103–11.
2. Kutteh WH. Recurrent pregnancy loss, in precis, an update in obstetrics and gynecology. Washington, DC: American College of Obstetrics and Gynecology; 2007.
3. Stephenson MD. Frequency of factors associated with habitual abortion in 197 couples. Fertil Steril 1996;66:24–9.
4. Jaslow CR, Carney JL, Kutteh WH. Diagnostic factors identified in 1020 women with two versus three or more recurrent pregnancy losses. Fertil Steril 2010; 93(4):1234–43.
5. Lund M, Kamper-Jørgensen M, Nielsen HS, et al. Prognosis for live birth in women with recurrent miscarriage: what is the best measure of success? Obstet Gynecol 2012;119:37–43.
6. Practice Committee of the American Society for Reproductive Medicine. Aging and infertility in women. Fertil Steril 2006;86(5 Suppl 1):S248–52.
7. Stirrat GM. Recurrent miscarriage. Lancet 1990;336:673–5.

8. Lathi RB, Gray Hazard FK, Heerema-McKenney A, et al. First trimester miscarriage evaluation. Semin Reprod Med 2011;29:463–9.
9. Nybo Andersen AM, Wohlfahrt J, Christens P. Maternal age and fetal loss: population based register linkage study. BMJ 2000;304:1708–12.
10. Harger JH, Archer DF, Marchese SG, et al. Etiology of recurrent pregnancy losses and outcome of subsequent pregnancies. Obstet Gynecol 1983;62: 574–81.
11. Quenby SM, Farquharson RG. Predicting recurring miscarriage: what is important? Obstet Gynecol 1993;82:132–8.
12. Roman E. Fetal loss rates and their relationship to pregnancy order. J Epidemiol Community Health 1984;38:29.
13. Hatasaka HH. Recurrent miscarriage: epidemiologic factors, definitions, and incidence. Clin Obstet Gynecol 1994;37:625–34.
14. Sugiura-Ogasawara M, Ozaki Y, Katano K, et al. Abnormal embryonic karyotype is the most frequent cause of recurrent miscarriage. Hum Reprod 2012;27: 2297–303.
15. Foyouzi N, Cedars MI, Huddleston HG. Cost-effectiveness of cytogenetic evaluation of products of conception in the patient with a second pregnancy loss. Fertil Steril 2012;98:151–5.
16. Bernardi LA, Plunkett BA, Stephenson MD. Is chromosome testing of the second miscarriage cost saving? A decision analysis of selective versus universal recurrent pregnancy loss evaluation. Fertil Steril 2012;98:156–61.
17. Stray-Pedersen B, Stray-Pedersen S. Etiologic factors and subsequent reproductive performance in 195 couples with a prior history of habitual abortion. Am J Obstet Gynecol 1984;148:140–6.
18. Jaslow CR, Kutteh WH. Effect of prior birth and miscarriage frequency on the prevalence of acquired and congenital uterine anomalies in women with recurrent miscarriage: a cross-sectional study. Fertil Steril 2013;99(7):1916–22.
19. Sugiura-Ogasawara M, Ozaki Y, Katano K, et al. Uterine anomaly and recurrent pregnancy loss. Semin Reprod Med 2011;29:514–21.
20. Stovall DW, Parrish SB, Van Voorhis BJ, et al. Uterine leiomyomas reduce the efficacy of assisted reproduction cycles: results of a matched follow-up study. Hum Reprod 1998;13:192–7.
21. Surrey ES, Lietz AK, Schoolcraft WB. Impact of intramural leiomyomate in patients with a normal endometrial cavity on in vitro fertilization-embryo transfer cycle outcome. Fertil Steril 2001;75:405–19.
22. American College of Obstetrics and Gynecologist. ACOG practice bulletin. Cervical insufficiency. Int J Gynaecol Obstet 2004;85:81–9.
23. Tuckerman E, Laird SM, Stewart R, et al. Markers of endometrial function in women with unexplained recurrent pregnancy loss. Hum Reprod 2004;19: 196–205.
24. Smith ML, Schust DJ. Endocrinology and recurrent early pregnancy loss. Semin Reprod Med 2011;29:482–90.
25. Cumming DC, Honore LH, Scott JZ, et al. The late luteal phase in infertile women: comparison of simultaneous endometrial biopsy and progesterone levels. Fertil Steril 1985;43:715–9.
26. Shepard MK, Senturia YD. Comparison of serum progesterone and endometrial biopsy for confirmation of ovulation and evaluation of luteal function. Fertil Steril 1977;28:541–8.
27. Goldstein P, Berrier J, Rosen S, et al. A meta-analysis of randomized control trials of progestational agents in pregnancy. BJOG 1989;96:265–74.

28. Haas DM, Ramsey PS. Progestogen for preventing miscarriage. Cochrane Database Syst Rev 2008;(2):CD003511.
29. Ghazeeri GS, Kutteh WH. Immunological testing and treatment in reproduction: frequency assessment of practice patterns at assisted reproduction clinics in the USA and Australia. Hum Reprod 2001;16:2130–5.
30. De Groot L, Abalovich M, Alexander EK, et al. Management of thyroid dysfunction during pregnancy and postpartum: an Endocrine Society clinical practice guideline. J Clin Endocrinol Metab 2012;97:2543–65.
31. Kutteh WH, Yetman DL, Carr AC, et al. Increased prevalence of antithyroid antibodies identified in women with recurrent pregnancy loss but not in women undergoing assisted reproduction. Fertil Steril 1999;71:843–8.
32. Mills JL, Simpson JL, Driscoll SG, et al. Incidence of spontaneous abortion among normal women and insulin-dependent diabetic women whose pregnancies were identified within 21 days of conception. N Engl J Med 1988;319:1617–23.
33. Sills ES, Perloe M, Palermo GD. Correction of hyperinsulinemia in oligoovulatory women with clomiphene-resistant polycystic ovary syndrome: a review of therapeutic rationale and reproductive outcomes. Eur J Obstet Gynecol Reprod Biol 2000;91:135–41.
34. Dlugi AM. Hyperprolactinemic recurrent spontaneous pregnancy loss: a true clinical entity or a spurious finding? [comment]. Fertil Steril 1998;70:253–5.
35. Hirahara F, Andoh N, Sawai K, et al. Hyperprolactinemic recurrent miscarriage and results of randomized bromocriptine treatment trials [comment]. Fertil Steril 1998;70:246–52.
36. Hofmann GE, Khoury J, Thie J. Recurrent pregnancy loss and diminished ovarian reserve. Fertil Steril 2000;74(6):1192–5.
37. Kutteh WH. Immunology of multiple endocrinopathies associated with premature ovarian failure. Endocrinologist 1996;6:462–6.
38. Franklin RD, Kutteh WH. Antiphospholipid antibodies (APA) and recurrent pregnancy loss: treating a unique APA positive population. Hum Reprod 2002;17:2981–5.
39. Kutteh WH, Lyda EC, Abraham SM, et al. Association of anticardiolipin antibodies and pregnancy loss in women with systemic lupus erythematosus. Fertil Steril 1993;60:449–55.
40. Miyakis S, Lockshin MD, Atsumi T, et al. International consensus statement on an update of the classification criteria for definite antiphospholipid syndrome (APS). J Thromb Haemost 2006;4:295–306.
41. Out HJ, Bruinse HW, Christians CM, et al. A prospective, controlled multicenter study of the obstetric risks of pregnant women with antiphospholipid antibodies. BJOG 1992;167:26–32.
42. Ernest JM, Marshburn PB, Kutteh WH. Obstetric antiphospholipid syndrome: an update on pathophysiology and management. Semin Reprod Med 2011;29:522–39.
43. Han CS, Mulla MJ, Brosens JJ, et al. Aspirin and heparin effect on basal and antiphospholipid antibody modulation of trophoblast function. Obstet Gynecol 2011;118(5):1021–8.
44. Rand JH. The antiphospholipid syndrome. Annu Rev Med 2003;54:409–24.
45. Di Simone N, Ferrazani S, Castellani R, et al. Heparin and low-dose aspirin restore placental human chorionic gonadotropin secretion abolished by antiphospholipid antibody containing sera. Hum Reprod 1997;12:2061–5.

46. Empson M, Lassere M, Craig JC, et al. Recurrent pregnancy loss with antiphospholipid antibody: a systematic review of therapeutic trials. Obstet Gynecol 2002;99:135–44.
47. Kutteh WH. Antiphospholipid antibody-associated recurrent pregnancy loss: treatment with heparin and low-dose aspirin is superior to low-dose aspirin alone. Am J Obstet Gynecol 1996;174:1584–9.
48. Pattison NS, Chamley LW, Birdsall M, et al. Does aspirin have a role in improving pregnancy outcome for women with the antiphospholipid syndrome? A randomized controlled trial. Am J Obstet Gynecol 2000;183:1008–12.
49. Ziakas PD, Pavlou M, Voulgarelis M. Heparin treatment in antiphospholipid syndrome with recurrent pregnancy loss: a systematic review and meta-analysis. Obstet Gynecol 2010;115(6):1256–62.
50. Mulla MJ, Brosens JJ, Chamley LW, et al. Antiphospholipid antibodies induce a pro-inflammatory response in first trimester trophoblast via the TLR4/MyD88 pathway. Am J Reprod Immunol 2009;62(2):96–111.
51. Committee on Practice Bulletins–Obstetrics, American College of Obstetricians and Gynecologists. Practice Bulletin No. 132: antiphospholipid syndrome. Obstet Gynecol 2012;120(6):1514–21.
52. Jablonowska B, Selbing A, Palfi M, et al. Prevention of recurrent spontaneous abortion by intravenous immunoglobulin: a double-blind placebo-controlled study. Hum Reprod 1999;14:838–41.
53. Stephenson MD, Kutteh WH, Purkiss S, et al. Intravenous immunoglobulin and idiopathic secondary recurrent miscarriage: a multicentered randomized placebo-controlled trial. Hum Reprod 2010;25(9):2203–9.
54. Coulam CB, Acacio B. Does immunotherapy for treatment of reproductive failure enhance live births? Am J Reprod Immunol 2012;67(4):296–304.
55. Scott JR. Immunotherapy for recurrent miscarriage. Cochrane Database Syst Rev 2003;(1):CD000112 [update of Cochrane Database Syst Rev. 2000;(2):CD000112; PMID: 10796135].
56. Laskin CA, Bombardier C, Hannah ME, et al. Prednisone and aspirin in women with autoantibodies and unexplained recurrent fetal loss. N Engl J Med 1997; 337:148–53.
57. Penta M, Lukic A, Conte MP, et al. Infectious agents in tissues from spontaneous abortions in the first trimester of pregnancy. New Microbiol 2003;26:329–37.
58. Lockwood C, Wendel G, Committee on Practice Bulletins–Obstetrics. Practice bulletin no. 124: inherited thrombophilias in pregnancy. Obstet Gynecol 2011; 118:730–40.
59. Hirshfeld-Cytron J, Sugiura-Ogasawara M, Stephenson MD. Management of recurrent pregnancy loss associated with a parental carrier of a reciprocal translocation: a systematic review. Semin Reprod Med 2011;29:470–81.
60. Hassold T, Chen N, Funkhouser J, et al. A cytogenetic study of 1000 spontaneous abortions. Ann Hum Genet 1980;44(Pt 2):151–78.
61. Werner M, Reh A, Grifo J, et al. Characteristics of chromosomal abnormalities diagnosed after spontaneous abortions in an infertile population. J Assist Reprod Genet 2012;29:817–20.
62. Nayak S, Pavone ME, Milad M, et al. Aneuploidy rates in failed pregnancies following assisted reproductive technology. J Womens Health (Larchmt) 2011; 20:1239–43.
63. Coulam CB, Goodman C, Dorfmann A. Comparison of ultrasonographic findings in spontaneous abortions with normal and abnormal karyotypes. Hum Reprod 1997;12:823–6.

64. Philipp T, Philipp K, Reiner A, et al. Embryoscopic and cytogenetic analysis of 233 missed abortions: factors involved in the pathogenesis of developmental defects of early failed pregnancies. Hum Reprod 2003;18:1724–32.

65. Mastenbroek S, Twisk M, van Echten-Arends J, et al. In vitro fertilization with preimplantation genetic screening. N Engl J Med 2007;357(1):9–17.

66. Practice Committee of Society for Assisted Reproductive Technology, Practice Committee of American Society for Reproductive Medicine. Preimplantation genetic testing: a practice committee opinion. Fertil Steril 2008;90:S136–43.

67. Harper JC, Wilton L, Traeger-Synodinos J, et al. The ESHRE PGD Consortium: 10 years of data collection. Hum Reprod Update 2012;18:234–47.

68. Forman EJ, Tao X, Ferry KM, et al. Single embryo transfer with comprehensive chromosome screening results in improved ongoing pregnancy rates and decreased miscarriage rates. Hum Reprod 2012;27:1217–22.

69. Schoolcraft WB, Fragouli E, Stevens J, et al. Clinical application of comprehensive chromosomal screening at the blastocyst stage. Fertil Steril 2010;94: 1700–6.

70. Brezina PR, Brezina DS, Kearns WG. Preimplantation genetic testing. BMJ 2012;345:e5908.

71. Wells D, Alfarawati S, Fragouli E. Use of comprehensive chromosomal screening for embryo assessment: microarrays and CGH. Mol Hum Reprod 2008;14:703–10.

72. Gardella JR, Hill JA 3rd. Environmental toxins associated with recurrent pregnancy loss. Semin Reprod Med 2000;18(4):407–24.

73. Harlap S, Shiono PH. Alcohol, smoking, and incidence of spontaneous abortions in the first and second trimester. Lancet 1980;2:173–8.

74. Kline J, Shroat P, Stein ZA, et al. Drinking during pregnancy and spontaneous abortion. Lancet 1980;2:176–80.

75. Andersen AM, Andersen PK, Olsen J, et al. Moderate alcohol intake during pregnancy and risk of fetal death. Int J Epidemiol 2012;41(2):405–13.

76. Ness RB, Grisso JA, Hrischinger N. Cocaine and tobacco use and the risk of spontaneous abortion. N Engl J Med 1999;340:333–9.

77. Johnson AR, Justin Milner J, Makowski L. The inflammation highway: metabolism accelerates inflammatory traffic in obesity. Immunol Rev 2012;249: 218–38.

78. Dlugosz L, Bracken MB. Reproductive effects of caffeine: a review and theoretical analysis. Epidemiol Rev 1992;4:83–100.

79. Yamazaki JN, Schull WJ. Perinatal loss and neurological abnormalities among children of the atomic bomb. Nagasaki and Hiroshima revisited, 1949 to 1989. JAMA 1990;264:605–9.

80. Brent RL. The effects of embryonic and fetal exposure to x-ray, microwaves, and ultrasound. Clin Perinatol 1986;13:615.

81. Brigham SA, Conlon C, Farquharson RG. A longitudinal study of pregnancy outcome following idiopathic recurrent miscarriage. Hum Reprod 1999;14: 2868–71.

82. Hyer JS, Fong S, Kutteh WH. Predictive value of the presence of an embryonic heartbeat for live birth: comparison of women with and without recurrent pregnancy loss. Fertil Steril 2004;82:1369–73.

Research Methodology in Recurrent Pregnancy Loss

Ole B. Christiansen, MD, DMSc[a,b,]*

KEYWORDS

- Recurrent pregnancy loss • Recurrent miscarriage • Medical research
- Research studies • Methodological flaws

KEY POINTS

- There is currently substantial disagreement concerning the diagnostic criteria for recurrent pregnancy loss (RPL), which renders comparisons between research studies in the area difficult.
- There are numerous methodological pitfalls that threaten the validity of research studies in the field of RPL and it is necessary for scientists and clinicians to be aware of them.
- Some of the methodological pitfalls are common for medical research in general, whereas some are specific for RPL research.
- Frequently seen methodological flaws in case-control studies are comparisons of biomarkers between patients with RPL and controls that differ from patients with regard to previous ongoing pregnancies, relevant endocrine factors, and viability of the fetal tissue at the time of sampling.
- In cohort studies, incomplete follow-up of patients in many studies has resulted in huge variations in estimates of the prognosis after RPL.
- Only a few small and heterogeneous double-blinded placebo-controlled trials of treatments of RPL have been carried out with very heterogeneous results.
- Proposals are given for improvements in the design of research studies in RPL that hopefully can improve the quality of studies in the future.

INTRODUCTION

Compared with the situation in other reproductive medicine disorders, such as tubal or male factor infertility and in other areas of medicine, there is very little consensus about which investigations are useful for identifying causes or estimating the prognosis and which treatments are effective in recurrent pregnancy loss (RPL). It is generally agreed that when the tubes are occluded, as diagnosed by laparoscopy or

[a] Fertility Clinic 4071, Copenhagen University Hospital Rigshospitalet, Blegdamsvej 9, DK-2100, Copenhagen, Denmark; [b] Department of Obstetrics and Gynecology, Aalborg University Hospital, Reberbansgade, DK-9000, Aalborg, Denmark
* Fertility Clinic 4071, Copenhagen University Hospital Rigshospitalet, Blegdamsvej 9, DK-2100, Copenhagen, Denmark.
E-mail address: olbc@rn.dk

Obstet Gynecol Clin N Am 41 (2014) 19–39
http://dx.doi.org/10.1016/j.ogc.2013.10.001
0889-8545/14/$ – see front matter © 2014 Elsevier Inc. All rights reserved.

hysterosalpingography (HSG), pregnancy can happen only after in vitro fertilization (IVF), and when the number of viable spermatozoa is very low, pregnancy can happen only after intracytoplasmatic sperm injection (ICSI). It is also generally agreed that IVF or ICSI are very efficient treatment methods for the 2 reproductive disorders. In recurrent early pregnancy loss there is much more disagreement about diagnosis, cause, and treatments. Although most guidelines from specialist societies do not support the screening of RPL women for hereditary thrombophilia factors or peripheral blood or endometrial natural killer (NK) cell numbers and function,[1–3] many clinics are still doing this, and whereas the Cochrane review[4] or national guidelines do not recommend immunotherapy[1,2] or preimplantation genetic screening (PGS)[5] for RPL, immunotherapy and PGS are still widely used in many clinics.

There could be many reasons why doctors very often do not adhere to the clinical guidelines regarding RPL:

- Pressure from desperate patients to do something although very few proven therapies really exist
- The doctors' economical motives, as many patients are desperate and willing to pay a lot of money for treatments that may provide them with some hope for a solution to their problem
- Current guidelines are based on few, small, and often poor-quality studies that cannot support strong, evidence-based recommendations

In this author's view, the third statement is the most important cause for this poor adherence to RPL guidelines. With regard to almost every diagnostic test or treatment for RPL, it is possible to find studies presenting data strongly in favor of this test or treatment and other studies strongly against. It is therefore often up to clinicians themselves to decide which studies they find trustworthy.

The aim of this article is to highlight pitfalls in research methodology that may explain why studies in RPL often provide very divergent results, and it is hoped that insight in this issue may help clinicians to decide which published studies are most valid. It may help researchers to eliminate methodological flaws in future studies, which may hopefully come to some kind of agreement about the usefulness of diagnostic tests and treatments in RPL.

CONTROVERSIES OF DEFINITION

It is disputed how to define RPL. It is important to realize that RPL is defined quite differently from most other diseases. Most diseases are defined by some unique pathoanatomical, clinical, or paraclinical findings being permanently present, whereas RPL is defined by a series of transient events in the past that may have be poorly registered.

The controversies concerning how to define RPL deal with

- The number of miscarriages needed for the diagnosis
- The role of nonconsecutive miscarriages
- The role of preclinical losses

Until 10 years ago, the definition of RPL was undisputedly 3 or more consecutive miscarriages, because it was commonly agreed that after 3 miscarriages the chance of live birth the next pregnancy without treatment was substantially decreased.[6] However, during the recent years, some national guidelines have adopted an RPL definition of only 2 clinically recognized miscarriages[1] or 2 not necessarily consecutive miscarriages.[7] This redefinition is based on finding similar frequencies of selected factors suggested to cause RPL: uterine abnormalities; antiphospholipid antibodies

(APL); parental chromosome aberrations; or the factor V Leiden mutation in women with 2, women with 3, and women with more miscarriages.[7,8] It is argued that when such risk factors already recommended in the screening of couples with 3 miscarriages can be found with similar prevalence in those with 2 miscarriages, they should also be examined in the latter. If the same tests are recommended in couples with 2 as well as those with 3 or more miscarriages, it is a short step to redefine RPL as 2 or more miscarriages. There is also now disagreement regarding which kind of pregnancy losses should be included in the criteria for RPL. Thirty years ago, because of the nonexistence of ultrasonic examinations and high sensitive pregnancy tests, pregnancies could not be diagnosed before gestational week (GW) 6 to 7; therefore, the pregnancy losses considered in the RPL diagnosis were miscarriages, which had normally been confirmed by curettage and histology. Pregnancies can now, owing to highly sensitive and specific β-human chorionic gonadotropin (hCG) tests, be diagnosed a few days after the due menstrual period, and many of these (biochemical pregnancies) will fail before it is possible to do transvaginal ultrasound. There is thus an urgent need to find a place for these kinds of losses in the RPL diagnosis. Because transiently positive pregnancy tests at the time of the due period are a frequent finding in women not using anticonception,[9] many gynecologists have been reluctant to include biochemical pregnancies in the RPL diagnosis, and the American Society for Reproductive Medicine (ASRM) definition of RPL (2 or more clinical miscarriages) completely disregards them.[1] A recent study from the European Society for Human Reproduction and Embryology (ESHRE) early pregnancy special interest group on the other side found that in patients with RPL, each early pregnancy loss confirmed only by a β-hCG test displays a negative prognostic impact equal to that of a clinical miscarriage, supporting the view that biochemical pregnancies should be included in the RPL diagnosis.[10] The different diagnostic criteria recommended in the national guidelines or by leading RPL clinics are[1,2,7,10] as follows:

- ≥3 consecutive pregnancy losses before 24 weeks of gestation
- ≥2 consecutive clinical pregnancy losses
- ≥3 consecutive clinical miscarriages and biochemical pregnancies
- ≥2 not necessarily consecutive pregnancy losses before 24 weeks of gestation

In numerous studies, it was found that the strongest predictive factor for new miscarriage in patients with RPL is the number of previous losses.[6,11] Because the same diagnosis, RPL, for the time being covers patients with a wide range of previous losses and therefore very different pregnancy prognoses, it will in the future be increasingly difficult to compare and combine different studies of outcome in patients with RPL (eg, results of randomized controlled trials [RCTs]). The only way to overcome this obstacle is that the investigators in such studies stratify the results according to the number of previous clinical miscarriages, as well as biochemical pregnancies or pregnancies of unknown location (PULs).

TYPES OF RESEARCH STUDIES

Different pitfalls characterize the 3 main types of research studies done in RPL:

- Case-control studies
- Cohort studies
- Intervention and treatment studies

For each category of studies, I provide an overview of the pitfalls that threaten the validity of the studies and the flaws often seen in publications: some of them can be seen in other areas of medical research and they are discussed superficially, whereas others that are specific for RPL research are discussed in more detail.

CASE-CONTROL STUDIES

Case-control studies always have a retrospective design. The frequency of a potential risk factor is investigated in a group of patients who have been sampled during a defined period (typically in a single clinic) with a specific disease diagnosis and compared with the corresponding frequency in a group of randomly selected individuals either without the disease or (if the disease is rare) selected from the background population. An estimate of the potential risk factors' association with the disease is typically given by the odds ratio (OR) with 95% confidence limits indicating the ratio between the frequency of the risk factor in diseased individuals and in controls.

Methodological errors in case-control studies can occur during the sampling of both patients and control subjects and errors can occur in the testing for potential risk factors.

Flaws in Sampling of Patients and Controls

Inconsistent diagnosis

The different definitions of RPL have already been discussed. Different RPL definitions will make comparisons between case-control studies originating from regions with different definitions increasingly difficult in the future.

Misclassification of disease/outcome status

Even if identical RPL definitions are used, patients in different studies can differ regarding the severity of the disease: the number of previous miscarriages. Because the RPL diagnosis is based on a series of past events, the validity of the diagnosis is dependent on the quality of the information that is available about these events. In many clinics, information about previous pregnancy losses comes primarily from interviewing the patients. Misclassification of disease/outcome status (the number of previous miscarriages) can be random or nonrandom. There are many examples of random outcome misclassification when dealing with miscarriages. Only 71% of miscarriages reported by women without RPL who have been treated at hospital could be verified in hospital records,[12] and in a retrospective study, 348 women recalled 30 (6%) of 507 miscarriages that were not reported in a prospective study several years before.[13] Random outcome misclassification results in an underestimate of the hypothesized association between exposure and disease/outcome in case-control studies (**Table 1**).

Retrospective information about previous pregnancy losses can also be subjected to nonrandom misclassification, also called recall or information bias. This misclassification is a difference in the ability or inclination to remember or report events or exposures in the past in individuals with or without particular characteristics. Women who had given birth to a child with a congenital malformation will search their memory extensively for any potentially teratogenic exposures during pregnancy and therefore retrospectively report more exposures than women who had delivered a healthy child, although there is no real difference in the frequency of harmful exposures in the 2 groups. Some women with 1 or 2 confirmed miscarriages will be more prone to interpret delayed menstruations or recall previous terminations as miscarriages than women without recent pregnancy losses, and thus erroneously get a diagnosis of RPL. Such nonrandom misclassification of disease/outcome status will result in either an overestimation or underestimation (see **Table 1**) of the true size of the hypothesized

Table 1
Important methodological pitfalls typical for research studies in RPL

Factor to Evaluate	Effect on Study Outcome
Definition of RPL ≤2 miscarriages	Decreases difference between risk variables in CCS and treatment effect in RCTs
Random misclassification	Decreases difference between risk variables in CCS
Nonrandom misclassification	Decreases or increases difference between risk variables in CCS or outcome variables in CS
Ascertainment bias	Increases difference between risk variables in CCS
Relevant mismatches between patients and controls	Increases difference between risk variables in CCS
Lack of protocol details/multiple testing	Overestimates significance of chance findings
Historical controls	Increases effects in treatment studies
Nonblinding	Increases or decreases treatment effects in RCTs
Premature termination after interim analysis	Decreases treatment effect in RCTs
Inclusion after detection of fetal heart action	Decreases treatment effect in RCTs
Poor characterization of RPL and subgroups of RPL	Renders comparisons between CCS and RCTs difficult and makes meta-analysis difficult
Unfounded exclusions of RCTs in systematic reviews	Bias combined risk estimates in meta-analyses

Abbreviations: CCS, case-control study; RCT, randomized controlled trial; RPL, recurrent pregnancy loss.

relationship between exposure and disease/outcome (RPL). To avoid random and nonrandom misclassification in RPL case-control studies, information about previous pregnancies should as much as possible be confirmed from external sources: records from hospitals, fertility clinics, and practitioners and serum hCG measurements should be documented from laboratory reports.

Ascertainment bias

In case-control studies, the frequency of a potential risk factor for the disorder under study (eg, RPL) is compared between patients and controls. Ascertainment or selection bias happens when patients with some clinical or paraclinical risk factor are preferentially referred to a specific clinic because of knowledge of the clinic's expertise or interest, and a study focusing on this particular risk factor is undertaken in the clinic. An example of ascertainment bias in RPL has been reported by Out and colleagues.[14] In this study, the frequency of the APLs anticardiolipin and lupus anticoagulant was higher in patients with RPL referred to a Dutch center for APL research than in controls. However, when patients with RPL with a history of thromboembolic or lupuslike symptoms were excluded, the prevalence of APL in the remaining patients with RPL did not differ from that of controls. The high prevalence of APL in the total group of patients resulted from the preferential referral of patients with RPL with APL-associated symptoms to the clinic due to its special expertise (see **Table 1**).

Ascertainment bias can also work in controls. In studies of risk factors for adverse pregnancy outcome, information is often obtained or blood samples drawn from women with healthy pregnancies coming for routine pregnancy control. Women giving informed consent to become controls are often better educated than average women, thereby decreasing the occurrence of lifestyle factors and exposures that may be harmful in pregnancy. When staff members or healthy blood donors are used as controls, these also undergo positive selection for being healthier than the average population.

Flaws in Estimating Risk Factors

Misclassification of exposure status

If the risk factor(s) under study is a potentially harmful exposure (eg, infection, smoking, medicamentation) in which the estimate of exposure is based on information retrospectively obtained from the patients and controls themselves; as previously discussed, this information can be subject to both random and nonrandom misclassification. If exposures have the same probability of being overreported/underreported in patients and controls, we are dealing with random misclassification and this will lead to an underestimate of the hypothesized relationship between exposure and disease/outcome. When the probability of exposure misclassification differs between patients and controls, nonrandom misclassification occurs. An example of nonrandom misclassification is when patients with RPL often recall an episode of fever during a pregnancy that subsequently failed, whereas controls with successful pregnancies report such episodes less often, although the incidence of fever in the 2 groups may be similar. Nonrandom misclassification of exposures can lead to an underestimate or overestimate of the true size of association between exposure and disease/outcome. To avoid misclassification in RPL case-control studies, data about exposures should be collected as much as possible from external sources: records from hospitals or practitioners or be collected before the outcome is known: in early pregnancy before miscarriage is diagnosed.

Confounding

In case-control studies, a confounding factor is a clinical or paraclinical factor that is associated with both the risk factor and the disease/outcome under study. If adequate measures are not taken, a confounding factor can be mistaken as a causal factor or diminish the estimate of the impact (OR) of the risk factor under study. In RPL studies, age is an important and common confounding factor. In studies of the prevalence of autoantibodies in patients with RPL and controls, age is associated with both the risk of miscarriage and RPL and the occurrence of autoantibodies. Elimination of the confounding effect of age during the inclusion phase of such studies can be undertaken by age-matching patients and controls and in the analysis phase by reporting autoantibody frequencies in different age strata of patients and controls and subsequently do adjustment by multivariate statistical methods.

Mismatch between patient and controls group

In case-control studies, the aim is to compare diseased and healthy individuals, which is quite straightforward regarding most diseases, but in RPL, research finding a suitable control group is a much more complex task (see **Table 1**; **Table 2**). Case-control studies in RPL research typically compare the following:

- Biomarkers in the blood or endometrium of nonpregnant women or in the blood of pregnant patients with RPL with the same biomarkers in women who do not have RPL
- Biomarkers in decidual or trophoblast tissue from women with RPL who have miscarried with the same biomarkers in tissue from non-RPL women who had an induced abortion.

Table 2
Suggested optimal control groups for the investigation of biomarkers in patients with RPL or their products of conception

| | Nongenetic Biomarkers | | | | | Genetic Biomarkers | |
| | Peripheral Blood | | Luteal Phase Endometrium | | Decidual/Trophoblast Tissue | | Peripheral Blood/Tissue | |
RPL^a	Controls^a	RPL^b	Controls^b	RPL^c	Controls^c	RPL	Controls
Primary/NP	Nulligravida/NP	Primary	Nulligravida	Primary, Euploid male embryo	Primary RPL Aneuploid embryo	All	Multipara
Secondary/NP	Previous birth/NP	Secondary	Previous birth	Secondary, Euploid male embryo	Secondary RPL Aneuploid embryo		
Primary GW5	Primigravida GW5						
Secondary GW5	Previous birth GW5						
Primary > GW6 Euploid male embryo	Primary RPL > GW6 Aneuploid embryo						
Secondary > GW6 Euploid male embryo	Secondary RPL > GW6 Aneuploid embryo						

In each double column, the suggested optimal controls are found to the right of the RPL column.

Abbreviations: GW, gestational week calculated from the first day of last menstrual period; NP, not pregnant; RPL, recurrent pregnancy loss.

a,b,c Women in each comparable pair should ideally have similar estrogen and progesterone levels in the nonpregnant state and similar hCG, estrogen, and progesterone levels in the pregnant state.

In studies of external exposures or genetic biomarkers, the ideal control group for patients with RPL is women with proven fertility: typically women with 2 or more uncomplicated births and no miscarriages, as genetic polymorphisms will not change according to reproductive history or be affected by endocrine factors or inflammation (see **Table 2**).

However, it is much more complex to identify the ideal controls for the investigation of nongenetically determined biomarkers in the blood, the endometrium, or trophoblast tissue. Some biomarkers, although exhibiting no impact on pregnancy outcome, may be different in patients with RPL and women with previous births merely because of their different reproductive histories.

An illustrative example is anti-HLA antibodies and studies of their role in RPL. Several years ago many articles reported that these antibodies could be detected much less frequently in the blood of patients with primary RPL (no previous ongoing pregnancies) than in control women who had previously given birth. It was postulated that lack of these "blocking antibodies" was a cause of the RPL and that deliberate immunization of the patients with paternal lymphocytes with the aim to stimulate antibody production would improve the pregnancy prognosis. It is now generally recognized that these antibodies are a common feature of normal ongoing pregnancy due to passage of fetal cells through the placenta into the maternal circulation during late pregnancy and they often persist for many years.[15] Therefore, it is not surprising that patients with primary RPL normally lack these antibodies, whereas multipara are often positive.

It has also been shown that cellular immunity is being permanently changed after a birth. Clones of cytotoxic lymphocytes with specificity for male-specific minor histocompatibility (HY) antigens develop in half of the women pregnant with a male fetus and the anti-HY cytotoxicity remains unchanged up to 18 years after delivery.[16] Long-term persistence of regulatory T cells[17] or/and persistence of fetal cells in the maternal circulation (fetal microchimerism) after a first ongoing pregnancy[18,19] may be the reason that most women remain immunologically tolerant to the fetus in spite of production of antibodies and lymphocytes with reactivity toward fetal antigens. The maternal immune system therefore recognizes many paternal/fetal alloantigens during an ongoing pregnancy and this very often induces permanent changes in immune reactivity to the fetus or trophoblast that may reside in lymphocytes carrying immunologic memory (memory T cells) in the peripheral blood, endometrium, or regional uterine lymph nodes. It is also possible, although much less studied, that transcription of messenger RNA (mRNA) and expression or production of proteins that are not related to the immune function (eg, receptors for hormones in the uterus, production of coagulation factors in the liver) can be permanently altered subsequent to the extensive physiologic changes taking place during a prior ongoing pregnancy (a pregnancy passing GW 22).

Because of these considerations, in RPL case-control studies controls should be matched to patients with RPL regarding a history of previous ongoing pregnancies (see **Table 2**). The ideal control group for patients with RPL who had never had an ongoing pregnancy would be women with repeated first trimester terminations due to social reasons; however, because this group is fortunately small, an alternative suitable control group would be women with no previous pregnancy. It may be argued that 1% of nulligravida would later experience RPL, but this small error is insignificant compared with the error associated with comparing nulliparous patients with RPL with multiparous controls. Patients with secondary RPL who had previously had a birth should of course be compared with controls with 1 previous live birth and no miscarriages.

Another factor that can confound case-control studies in RPL research and should be adjusted for as much as possible is differences in hormones relating to reproduction and pregnancy. Many factors relating to immune function (eg, cytokines) and the coagulation system (eg, proteins C and S) are influenced by estrogen and progesterone levels.[20] The level of expression of a series of cytokine mRNA in endometrial cells increases markedly from the follicular to the late secretory phase, probably influenced by cyclic changes of estrogen and progesterone.[21] It has been shown that lymphocytes that can induce immunologic tolerance (regulatory T cells) are attracted to the feto-maternal interface by hCG produced by the trophoblast,[22] which may have profound importance for measurements of immune biomarkers in the uterus during pregnancy. Because concentrations of hCG, estrogens, progesterone, cortisone, and pregnancy-associated placental protein A (PAPP-A) change markedly according to menstrual cycle phase or progressing gestation, the level of biomarkers affected by hormones is dependent on phase of menstrual cycle or time of gestation. Therefore, as a main rule, nongenetic biomarkers should be investigated in patients with RPL and controls matched by menstrual cycle phase in nonpregnant women and length of gestation during pregnancy (see **Table 2**).

A further problem arises when biomarkers in the blood or uterus, which are affected by hormones, are investigated in patients with RPL just before or at the time of miscarriage and compared with similar measurements in controls with a healthy ongoing pregnancy. Most of the pregnancy-related hormones, hCG, estrogen, and PAPP-A, decrease in threatened miscarriage and finding differences in a specific biomarker between women with a miscarriage or a healthy pregnancy, respectively, may be severely confounded by the fact that hormones in the former group are lower than in the control group.

A last but important factor that may confound case-control studies in RPL research is differences in the viability and inflammatory status of the uterine content before or at the time of miscarriage in patients and at the time of induced abortion in controls. At the time of embryonic death, the trophoblast will undergo necrosis and intrauterine hemorrhage will often induce inflammation in the decidual tissue, which can be reflected in measurements of immunologic biomarkers in the blood or decidual/trophoblast tissue. In contrast, the same biomarkers in the blood of controls with an ongoing normal pregnancy or in the blood or decidual/trophoblast tissue from controls with an induced abortion on social indication will not be influenced by inflammation. Unfortunately, in many publications, levels of biomarkers associated with immune function or apoptosis (programed cell death) in the blood or decidual/trophoblast tissue are compared between women with a missed abortion and women with a normal ongoing pregnancy or women undergoing induced abortion. In many of these publications, finding differences in levels of such biomarkers are interpreted as proof that changes in maternal immune reactions or apoptosis are causing miscarriage or RPL. To avoid detecting biomarkers in patients with RPL that differ from those in controls merely due to processes being a result of rather than a cause of miscarriage, measurements in peripheral blood should be undertaken in very early pregnancy (eg, GW 5) at a time when the feto-placental unit is very tiny and not expected to affect systemic inflammatory responses and before the confounding effect of declining hormones in patients take place (see **Table 2**).[23]

Another approach to counteract the methodological problem associated with the comparison of necrotic and vital tissue is to do karyotyping of embryos from missed abortions in women with or without RPL. Biomarkers in the blood or decidual/trophoblast tissue can then be compared between patients with euploid male embryos (to avoid erroneous karyotyping of maternal tissue) and patients with embryos with a chromosome abnormality that definitively will cause early embryonic death. Levels of biomarkers that are influenced by embryonic and trophoblast necrosis and inflammation may be equally affected in women with euploid and aneuploid miscarriages. Therefore, differences in expression of biomarkers between the women/embryos from the 2 groups can probably be attributed to factors that may have caused euploid miscarriage. Examples of such studies that point to a causal role of inflammatory cytokines in RPL is the study by Calleja-Agius and colleagues,[24] finding significantly higher plasma tumor necrosis factor-α, interferon-γ, interleukin (IL)-6, and IL-10 levels in women with euploid miscarriages than in healthy pregnancy, whereas these cytokines were not increased in women with aneuploid miscarriages. Another study similarly found increased numbers of activated leucocytes in RPL women with a miscarriage with an euploid compared an aneuploid embryo.[25]

As illustrated previously, finding a suitable control group for measurement of nongenetically determined biomarkers is a difficult task. Adherence to the recommendations given previously (see **Table 2**) may diminish the risk of conducting a case-control study that is methodologically flawed but offers no guarantee. The factors that should not differ between cases and controls in RPL research are the following:

- Number of previous ongoing pregnancies
- Levels of estrogen and progesterone in nonpregnant women
- Levels of estrogen, progesterone, and hCG in pregnant women
- Degree of viability of decidual or trophoblast tissue

I realize that very few case-control studies in RPL meet these criteria, especially the criteria of similar hormonal levels. More research should be done regarding genetically determined biomarkers because these are robust to the confounding effects discussed in this section. It is possible that some nongenetic biomarkers may also be robust to the effects of the mentioned confounding factors (eg, reproductive hormones). However, only when it has been proven in separate studies that a specific factor (eg, hormone) is not affecting the biomarker under study, a confounding effect of the factor can be ignored in subsequent case-control studies.

Lack of Protocol Data or a Priory Hypothesis

As a referee, I have often discovered that some research groups have published a series of case-control studies in different articles often in different journals, each case-control study dealing with only one specific biomarker, which was found to be significantly increased in patients with RPL. When the articles are carefully read and the data compared it seems that all the biomarkers have been investigated in the same patient and control groups in the same period. In the articles, no information was given about how many biomarkers were investigated in each study and what was the a priori hypothesis. The suspicion is that in many of these studies, the investigators have tested a huge series of biomarkers using a multiplex testing panel that can test for hundreds of (often genetic) biomarkers in 1 day and they report only data of those biomarkers that (by chance) are found significantly increased in RPL. After this "fishing expedition," the biomarkers being significantly associated with RPL are published one by one in separate articles according to the "salami method" without providing any information about how many biomarkers were investigated. In this way, the investigators can expand their publication list in an easy way. This "disguised multiple testing" is a maligned design, because the referees of the articles have no chance to know that multiple testing was done and to ask the investigators to do the appropriate statistical adjustment (see later in this article) and modify the conclusions. In the more benign cases, the investigators openly provide details of all tested biomarkers/variables in tables and the referees can then ask for adjustment if not already done.

This illustrates the problem that in many studies (especially case-control studies) dealing with RPL and other disorders, it is often unclear whether the result being reported as the main finding really was part of the a priori hypothesis from the start or whether it was a finding discovered during the conduct of the study: a post hoc finding (see **Table 1**).

As a preventive measure, high-ranking journals request the investigators to give more details of the study protocols or the protocols should be available on an online public registry (www.ClinicalTrials.Gov) before the beginning of the study. All journals should, as a minimum, request the investigators in the "materials and methods" section to provide information from the study protocol about the a priori hypothesis, main outcome measures, and sample size calculations, and to list all risk factors and biomarkers that were planned to test and actually tested.

Multiple Testing

Most case-control studies in RPL can be categorized as discovery studies in which there is no prior hypothesis about which associations are probable and therefore a series of biomarkers are investigated openly or disguised. Testing of multiple biomarkers is facilitated by the introduction of multiplex testing panels that can test hundreds of biomarkers at a time, thereby reducing the costs immensely. If, for example, 40 different biomarkers are tested in patients and controls and a P value for significance of less than .05 was chosen, it is expected that 2 ($40 \times 0.05 = 2$) biomarkers will be significantly increased or decreased in patients merely by chance. If no a priori hypothesis about which biomarker was the primary focus of the study was made (discovery study) the P values for all tested biomarkers should be subject to the Bonferroni adjustment by multiplying the P value with the number of comparisons made. If 1 or 2 biomarkers are still significantly associated with RPL after this adjustment, the association must be confirmed in at least 1 independent study (replication study) with the a priori hypothesis that the variables are associated with RPL.

Interpretation

Causality can rarely, if ever, be stated after finding a potential risk factor statistically significantly associated with a disease. According to Bradford-Hill criteria,[26] there are several demands for stating causality, the most important being the following:

- The criterion of temporality: that the risk factor occurs before the occurrence of the disease.
- The criterion of a biologic gradient: there should be a positive correlation between the severity of a putative risk factor and the severity of the disorder.

In studies of RPL, the first criterion can be documented only in prospective studies finding that the presence of a potential risk factor increases the risk of a new miscarriage compared with its absence. In RPL, the other criterion can be documented if there is a correlation between the severity of a potential risk factor, for example, concentration of APL antibody, and the severity of RPL = number of miscarriages in the patients. Findings in some previously quoted studies may indeed be interpreted as evidence against the investigated variables being causative for RPL because no biologic gradient was discovered.[7,8]

COHORT STUDIES

As stated in the previous section: to document that an exposure found to be associated with RPL in a case-control study is indeed a causal factor for RPL, a prospective study is needed.

A prospective study is normally designed as a cohort study. A group of individuals positive and another group of individuals negative for the exposure/potential risk factors for the disease (outcome) are identified. These 2 groups are now called cohorts and they are observed during a defined time period in which the occurrence of the outcome under study is monitored in the cohorts.

Concurrent Versus Nonconcurrernt Cohorts

In concurrent cohort studies, individuals assigned to the 2 cohorts are followed prospectively, whereas in nonconcurrent (or retrospective) cohort studies, the assignment to the cohorts is done on the basis of the detection of an exposure at a time in the past when the outcome under study had not yet happened. If the disease under study is RPL, such a concurrent cohort study could ideally assign 20-year-old women who had not yet been pregnant and who have been tested for relevant biomarkers into a hereditary thrombophilia positive and negative cohort. These 2 cohorts are then followed until the women had aged 45 years and the occurrence of RPL in the 2 cohorts is registered and compared between the cohorts. Adjustment for other risk factors for RPL, such as age at the first pregnancy attempt, body mass index (BMI), and so forth, should be undertaken in a multivariate analysis. It is clear that such a cohort study will probably never be undertaken; because of the low frequency of RPL, tens of thousands of women must be included and followed for 25 years: nobody would have the resources for that. Instead cohort studies focusing on pregnancy outcome after a diagnosis of RPL will be a easier task to perform. Still, concurrent cohort studies can take many years and therefore almost all cohort studies of patients with RPL have been nonconcurrent. To give an example, my group investigated hereditary thrombophilia factors (factor II and factor V Leiden mutations) in the patients referred to the RPL clinic in Denmark between 1986 and 2008, in 62% of the cases using DNA, which was stored but not tested for the thrombophilia-associated mutations before after the outcome of the first pregnancy after referral had been registered.[27] In most cases, the patients and their doctors were therefore unaware of the exposure status at the time of the first pregnancy after referral and none of the patients received anticoagulation treatment. In a good nonconcurrent cohort study, information about both exposure and outcome status should not be available at the time the cohorts are formed. The patients were thus in a nonconcurrent (retrospective) cohort study assigned to a hereditary thrombophilia positive and negative cohort, and outcome of the first pregnancy after referral to the clinic was "outcome." In a logistic regression analysis, adjusting for the impact of number of previous pregnancy losses, maternal age, and smoking, it was found that the presence of the hereditary thrombophilia factors significantly decreased the OR for birth in the first subsequent pregnancy (OR = 0.48, $P = .05$) compared with their absence. Thus, a much easier approach than doing a large concurrent cohort study can provide results documenting the importance of potential causal factors in RPL.

Nonrandom Misclassification

Cohort studies are prone to methodological errors, which are important to recognize when conducting or assessing them. Nonrandom misclassification is a significant threat to the validity of cohort studies; however, unlike case-control studies in which the patients or controls are the main source of the erroneous information leading to misclassification, in cohort studies it is the researchers who are responsible. In occupational medicine, workers are exposed to substances thought to increase the risk for some disease. Because of that knowledge, these workers are often monitored more closely than nonexposed workers and symptoms of disease (outcome) may be registered more often in the exposed than in the nonexposed cohort. Biased intensity of monitoring is also a problem in reproductive medicine research. In a cohort study of women with obesity (the exposure) or no obesity, to investigate whether obesity increases the risk of miscarriage, many obese women will have polycystic ovary syndrome (PCOS) and anovulation and therefore undergo assisted reproductive technology (ART) treatment, whereas most nonobese women will be able to conceive without the need of ART. In ART cycles, a β-hCG test is normally done 14 days after ovulation or embryo transfer, and all biochemical pregnancies will be detected, whereas among non-ART patients, they will often remain undetected. Therefore such a cohort study may show that obese women have an increased risk of pregnancy loss but this may be a result of nonrandom misclassification of the outcome.

In RPL cohort studies, misclassification is also a significant problem. The prognosis after a diagnosis of RPL is heavily disputed: various prospective studies have reported the chance of live birth in the first pregnancy after referral in patients with 3 miscarriages to be between 63% and 87%, with 4 miscarriages between 44% and 73%, and with 5 miscarriages between 25% and 52%, respectively.[11] These very different estimates are frustrating: for a patient with RPL, it is of utmost importance to know whether her chance for live birth is 44% or 73%. This variation may be caused by random misclassification within individual studies. Data from 2 placebo-controlled trials of intravenous immunoglobulin (Ivlg) conducted in Sweden[28] and Denmark,[29] respectively, may clarify the issue. Patients with 3 or more miscarriages who met the inclusion criteria for participation in the trials were encouraged to conceive and call the clinics as soon as they got pregnant. When the Swedish trial (cohort 1) was concluded after 4 years, 50.6% of the patients were classified as not having achieved pregnancy, only 3.4% had pre-embryonic losses, and 10.1% had embryonic losses (**Fig. 1**). When the Danish trial (cohort 2) was concluded after 6 years, only 14.7% did not report pregnancy, 22.4% had pre-embryonic losses, and 27.9% had embryonic losses. When live birth rates in cohorts 1 and 2 are calculated with the number of recognized pregnancies in the denominator, they become 72.7% and 44.8%, respectively (P<.005). The most striking difference between the 2 cohorts is the very much higher frequency of nonconception in cohort 1 than in cohort 2. This may be because of the simple fact that the Danish patients were told that they could not be included in the trial if they contacted the clinic more than

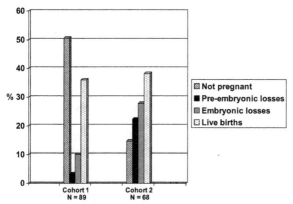

Fig. 1. Classification of pregnancy outcome in 4 categories of patients with RPL eligible for participation in a Swedish (cohort 1) and a Danish (cohort 2) placebo-controlled trial of Ivlg. In each cohort, patients receiving Ivlg and placebo are combined.

5 days after the missed menstrual period, whereas in the Swedish trial, patients were included only when fetal heart action could be demonstrated in GW 6 to 7. In cohort 2, every conception was probably registered, whereas in cohort 1, many pre-embryonic losses may have been misclassified as nonconception. Another published cohort of patients with RPL that estimated the chance of live birth in the first subsequent pregnancy, also found that 30% of the patients reported no further pregnancies after referral to the clinic or were lost to follow-up.[30] This is again a much higher frequency that the 14.7% in the Danish cohort. As in the Swedish cohort, this difference is probably caused by incomplete follow-up resulting in misclassification of preclinical pregnancy losses as nonconception. When results from different cohort studies are compared, this misclassification becomes nonrandom (see **Table 1**).

Cohorts Estimating Live Births Per Time Unit

The aforementioned examples illustrate the unreliability of studies of RPL cohorts based on the patients' self-reporting of outcome of the first subsequent pregnancy. My group has therefore proposed a more robust method of estimating the prognosis for the patients. We obtained information about subsequent live birth from the national birth registry (which registers 100% of all births in Denmark) for all patients with RPL referred to our clinic from 1986 to 2008. We could then calculate age-specific and prior number of miscarriages–specific proportions of patients who had achieved a live birth within 5 and 15 years after the first consultation (66.7% and 71.1%, respectively).[11] Such an estimate with the rate of live birth in the numerator and the observation time in the denominator is a robust and clinical relevant way to estimate the prognosis, and it is not sensitive to the intensity of monitoring as in the previously discussed methods. However, it can, of course, be used only in countries with a complete and valid national birth registration system. Our estimates of the long-term live birth rates in subsets of patients with RPL, most of whom had attempted pregnancy several times after referral, are generally lower than those reported in the first pregnancy in a frequently quoted cohort,[30] and because our cohort is not sensitive to misclassification, the other cohort probably provides too optimistic rates.

TREATMENT TRIALS

In a time of embracement of evidence-based medicine, all treatments, new as well as established, should undergo testing in clinical trials. With regard to RPL, clinical treatment trials compare miscarriage rates in patients with RPL given one specific treatment in the present pregnancy compared with outcome in a control group not receiving the treatment.

Historical Controls

In some treatment trials, pregnancy outcome in a group of patients treated in the present was compared with outcome in nontreated controls from the past, so-called historical controls.

In a small study of PGS in the treatment of RPL in women aged 35 years,[31] the live birth rate after PGS was for each patient compared with the expected rate in women with similar age and number of miscarriages calculated from a historical cohort.[30] The investigators found that the live birth rate after PGS was higher than the expected rate using the data from the historical cohort. Comparing outcome in contemporary RPL patient groups with historical control groups carries a substantial risk of producing unreliable results (see **Table 1**). It is extremely difficult to be sure that a group of patients with RPL identified in the past is comparable with a present group, as ascertainment of patients, screening methods, and pregnancy-monitoring procedures have changed substantially with time.

A variant of the use of historical controls is the use of the treated patients as their own controls. In RPL research, the live birth rate in patients with RPL before a specific intervention is compared with the birth rate after the intervention. The use of this method is still seen in publications especially concerning surgical treatment of RPL, but also regarding other treatment modalities, such as metformin.[32] Although using the patients as their own controls at a first glance would appear ideal, this method is severely flawed due to the phenomenon *regression to the mean*.[33] The population of patients with RPL may comprise the following:

- A subset of women who have experienced the miscarriages merely because of chance (repeated embryonic aneuploidies) with a low intrinsic risk of miscarriage in each pregnancy but the women have been sampled asymmetrically from a binominal distribution.
- A subset of women with maternal risk factors with a higher intrinsic risk of miscarriage.

In the former subset, on any subsequent measure (new pregnancy) the mean risk of miscarriage will be closer to the (low) mean of the original population in spite of no intervention due to *regression to the mean*. If they are selected to a treatment trial, the chance of success in the next pregnancy will be excellent in spite of no intervention. In a trial of cerclage, the posttreatment birth rate was statistically significantly higher than before cerclage and it was concluded that cerclage increases the live birth rate. However, using this method, all types of interventions can be proved to be efficient in the treatment of RPL, even placebo.[34] In an RCT of infusion of allogeneic lymphocytes versus placebo in RPL, the patients who received placebo had a live birth rate of 12.5% before they entered the trial and subsequently 47.7% gave birth after placebo infusions. By comparing birth rates before and after placebo by χ^2 test, the statistics claim that placebo is highly efficient in treating RPL. This apparent, but false, improvement of outcome can be completely attributed to the effect of *regression to the mean*.

Randomized Controlled Trials

Proper evaluation of treatments in RPL can be done only in RCTs. In RCTs, patients are prospectively allocated to treatment or no-treatment or placebo by some randomization procedure that cannot be influenced by the researcher. This will increase the chance that confounding variables, which can influence the prognosis, are equally distributed in the groups.

Blinding

In the ideal RCT, allocation to active treatment or a placebo that cannot be distinguished from each other is undertaken according to a randomization list so that the trial is blinded (masked) for both the researchers and patients, a so-called double-blind design. The effects of blinding in RCTs are as follows:

- Blinding of the doctors will ensure the same monitoring and concomitant therapy in both groups
- Blinding of the patients will provide them with the full placebo effect that due to neuroendocrine pathways may exhibit a positive effect on pregnancy outcome in RPL[35]
- Blinding of the patients will diminish the dropout rate and associated poor registration of subsequent outcome in those allocated to the expected less-efficient treatment

Several RCTs in the RPL area are unfortunately not blinded. None of the trials testing the effect of heparin plus low-dose aspirin in patients with RPL with or without APL has compared this intervention against a placebo for heparin but only against low-dose aspirin alone or a peroral placebo for aspirin.[36–38] This is probably due to the reluctance to use a placebo drug for daily subcutaneous injections during the whole period of pregnancy. Although the outcome in RPL, a new miscarriage, can be determined by objective methods that are not impacted by blinding/nonblinding, nonblinding can negatively or positively influence outcome (see **Table 1**) in the groups receiving nontreatment or expected less-efficient treatment compared with the expected more-efficient treatment (tablets vs injections plus tablets).

Although a double-blinded randomized placebo-controlled trial is the best design to obtain valid data concerning treatment effect, this method does not guarantee that the results are trustworthy, as other circumstances can confound or weaken the results.

Confounding in RCTs

Most RCTs in RPL have included a small number of patients and this increases the risk that a confounding variable, such as number of prior miscarriages and age, by chance is unevenly distributed between the 2 allocation groups. In a small RCT, it is not sufficient to show that the mean number of previous miscarriages or age is not statistically significantly different in the 2 allocation groups; these variables can still significantly confound the results. The best way to counteract uneven distribution of prognostic variables in RCTs is by doing block-randomization, whereby separate allocation of patients is done according to groups with comparable number of miscarriages and age.

Inclusion after GW 6

In numerous RCTs, patients with RPL have been allocated and included in the trial only when an ultrasonographic examination has demonstrated a viable intrauterine pregnancy in GW 6 to 7.[28,38,39] This design can unfortunately substantially diminish any effect of the active intervention (see **Table 1**). Twenty-two percent of closely monitored patients with RPL have pre-embryonic losses (see **Fig. 1**), which comprise almost half of all their pregnancy losses.[29] When treatment in RCTs starts only after the demonstration of fetal heart action, almost half of the risk period for miscarriage has thus passed and the spontaneous prognosis at that time is good.[40] Therefore, very large numbers of participants are needed to show any treatment effect. Furthermore, when treatment is started only in GW 6 to 7, the pregnancy has been exposed to the full harmful effect of thrombophilic or immunologic factors for 2 to 3 weeks before initiation of the potential beneficial therapy. The trophoblast or fetus, although viable at that time, may have suffered irreversible damage that cannot be counteracted by initiating active therapy.

Premature discontinuation of an RCT

In many RCTs, at least 1 interim analysis is performed during the conduct of the trial and it is prematurely stopped if the results at this analysis show that a statistically significant effect of the intervention could not be obtained even if the trial was continued until the originally planned number of participants was reached. Many RCTs in the area of RPL have been stopped prematurely after performance of an interim analysis,[28,41,42] and this poses a substantial problem in interpreting the results, especially when they are included in systematic reviews and meta-analyses. There is a great risk that the difference between the outcome in the intervention and nonintervention/placebo groups at the stopping point after the interim analysis due to a random fluctuation is smaller than if the trial had been continued to the planned number of participants; if the difference had been larger the trial had been allowed to continue. RCTs stopped after interim analyses will therefore be expected to report intervention effects that are smaller than the true effects (see **Table 1**) and, if included in systematic reviews, their scientific quality should accordingly be down-graded.

Inclusion of several outcomes from the same patient

In case series and RCTs in RPL research, several pregnancy outcomes from the same patients are sometimes included.[43,44] This is a methodological flaw, as the outcomes of pregnancies in individual patients with RPL due to the importance of maternal risk factors (eg, age, number of prior losses) are linked variables. The commonly used statistical methods, such as χ^2 test and Fisher test, require that the tested variables are independent and cannot be used. Therefore, only one pregnancy outcome from each patient should be included in trials testing interventions, whether randomized or not.

Systematic Reviews

A systematic review is a review that uses systematic and explicit methods to critically appraise a research topic; statistical methods such as meta-analyses may be used to analyze and summarize the results of the included studies. Both case-control studies and RCTs can be subject to such reviews and their results are considered the highest level of evidence. In RPL research, systematic reviews have in particular focused on intervention/treatment studies. The pooled OR calculated from the combination of results in the meta-analysis is considered a good measure for the overall effect of the intervention/treatment under study. However, because most treatments exhibit different effects in different subsets of patients (eg, men and women or patients with severe vs less severe disease), an important use of meta-analyses is to identify subgroups of patients who have the largest benefit of treatment.[45] I focus my discussion regarding systematic reviews in RPL on those dealing with immunotherapy with IvIg, because these reviews have included the largest numbers of studies and patients and the discussion illustrates the pitfalls and methodological flaws that characterize systematic reviews in the area of RPL treatment. Four different systematic reviews have been published concerning IvIg treatment in RPL,[4,42,46,47] which have provided very different results and conclusions. This variability is in my view caused by either (1) a failure to recognize the need of doing separate analysis in relevant subgroups of patients or (2) by unfounded exclusions of RCTs in the systematic reviews. A Cochrane review[4] did not find any difference in live birth rate between IvIg and placebo in all included patients with RPL but made no distinction between patients with primary and secondary RPL, which would be relevant, as 2 published trials had found the IvIg efficient exclusively in the latter group.[29,48] In contrast, another systematic review based on almost the same patients recognized the relevance of doing this subgroup analysis and found the live birth rate significantly higher in IvIg-treated than in placebo-treated patients with secondary RPL.[46]

The 2 most recent systematic reviews on IvIg in RPL included only patients with "unexplained" RPL, which meant that trials that had included patients with RPL positive for APL according to the assays used in the individual clinics and according to the local cutoff values were excluded.[42,47] The investigators considered that 2 RCTs included APL-positive patients and all 92 patients in these RCTs were completely excluded from the systematic reviews comprising 25.3% of all 364 patients with RPL participating in RCTs of IvIg. Exclusion of this substantial proportion of all randomized patients with RPL appears to be an enormous waste of valid information. In one of the excluded RCTs, none of the patients in fact had APL and in the other almost all patients who tested APL-positive had very low titers.[49] Only 3% would be considered APL-positive according to the current criteria.[50] On the other hand, an RCT that was not excluded did in fact include APL-positive patients[51] and several of the other RCTs did not report details of APL assays or cutoff levels. Because both excluded RCTs had found a substantial effect of IvIg in patients with secondary RPL, doing the meta-analyses without these resulted in the conclusion in both systematic reviews that there is no benefit of IvIg either in primary or secondary RPL.[42,47] As stated by my group and others, we find the methodology of these systematic reviews questionable and without the exclusions it can be proved that IvIg is indeed efficient in secondary RPL.[49,52] As previously mentioned, it is legal and desirable to do meta-analyses in subgroups of patients to identify subgroups that benefit best from treatment, and such a subgroup could be patients with RPL without APL. However, a systematic review excluding these patients should of course exclude only those patients who are positive for APL and not complete RCTs with only a tiny minority of participants being APL-positive. Furthermore, in most published relevant RCTs, insufficient information is given about the APL assays and cutoff values, which may vary substantially between the trials. To carry out a meta-analysis of therapies in APL-negative patients with RPL based on good research methodology, it is therefore necessary to collect data on APL levels for each included patient. In most cases, these data on individual patients can be obtained only by contacting the investigators of the RCTs. If such a collection of raw data is not done, the resulting systematic review and meta-analysis will produce biased results.

This discussion illustrates that even conclusions from systematic reviews should be evaluated critically and a systematic review is not per se the highest level of evidence. If they are not conducted according to rigorous and systematic rules, they will end up being no more evidence-based than the narrative reviews of the old days (see **Table 1**).

SUMMARY

Most causes of RPL are poorly elucidated and may have a more multifactorial etiology than infertility and in many instances the cause-effect relationship is unclear. Furthermore, the RPL population is much smaller that the infertile population, thereby making it difficult to conduct studies with adequate statistical power.

These problems render research in RPL inherently difficult and only methodologically high-quality studies are expected to produce useful results. Unfortunately, such high-quality research studies are rare in the area of RPL.

All types of studies in RPL research are characterized by methodological pitfalls, which are often not recognized by the researchers or readers. Failure to recognize these can completely invalidate studies in the area. It is hoped that this review, by setting focus on the problem, can help improve studies in the area of RPL in the future.

REFERENCES

1. The Practice Committee of the American Society for Reproductive Medicine. Evaluation and treatment of recurrent pregnancy loss: a committee opinion. Fertil Steril 2012;98:1103–11.
2. Royal College of Obstetricians and Gynaecologists. The investigation and treatment of couples with recurrent first-trimester and second-trimester miscarriage. RCOG Green-top Guideline No. 17. 2011.
3. Jauniaux E, Farquharson RG, Christiansen OB, et al. Evidence-based guidelines for the investigation and medical treatment of recurrent miscarriage. Hum Reprod 2006;21:2216–22.

4. Porter TF, LaCoursiere Y, Scott JR. Immunotherapy for recurrent miscarriage. Cochrane Database Syst Rev 2006;(2):CD000112. http://dx.doi.org/10.1002/14651858.
5. The Practice Committee of the Society for Assisted Reproductive Technology, Practice committee of the American Society for Reproductive Medicine. Preimplantation genetic testing: a Practice Committee opinion. Fertil Steril 2008;90: S136–46.
6. Nybo Andersen AM, Wohlfart J, Christens P, et al. Maternal age and fetal loss: population based register linked study. BMJ 2000;320:1708–12.
7. van den Boogaard E, Cohn DM, Korevaard JC, et al. Number and sequence of preceding miscarriages and maternal age for the prediction of antiphospholipid syndrome in women with recurrent miscarriage. Fertil Steril 2013;99:188–92.
8. Jaslow CR, Careney JL, Kutteh WH. Diagnostic factors identified in 1020 women with two versus three or more recurrent pregnancy losses. Fertil Steril 2010;193: 1234–43.
9. Wilcox AJ, Weinberg CR, O'Connor JF, et al. Incidence of early loss of pregnancy. N Engl J Med 1988;319:189–94.
10. Kolte AM, van Oppenraaij RH, Quenby S, et al. Biochemical pregnancy loss and pregnancy of unknown location are prognostically important for unexplained recurrent miscarriage. Under review.
11. Lund M, Kamper-Jørgensen M, Nielsen HS, et al. Prognosis for live birth in women with recurrent miscarriage. What is the best measure of success? Obstet Gynecol 2012;119:37–43.
12. Axelsson G, Rylander R. Validation of questionnaire reported miscarriage, malformation and birth weight. Int J Epidemiol 1984;13:94–8.
13. Wilcox AJ, Horney LF. Accuracy of spontaneous abortion recall. Am J Epidemiol 1984;120:727–33.
14. Out HJ, Bruinse HW, Christiaens GC, et al. A prospective, controlled multicenter study on the obstetric risks of pregnant women with antiphospholipid antibodies. Am J Obstet Gynecol 1992;167:26–32.
15. Regan L, Braude PR, Hill DP. A prospective study of the incidence, time of appearance and significance of anti-paternal lymphocytotoxic antibodies in human pregnancy. Hum Reprod 1991;6:294–8.
16. Lissauer D, Piper K, Goodyear O, et al. Fetal-specific CD8+ cytotoxic T cell responses develop during normal human pregnancy and exhibit broad functional capacity. J Immunol 2012;189:1072–80.
17. Wegienka G, Havstad S, Bobbitt KR, et al. Within-woman change in regulatory T cells from pregnancy to the postpartum period. J Reprod Immunol 2011;88: 58–65.
18. Gamill HS, Guthrie KA, Aydelotte TM, et al. Effect of parity on fetal and maternal microchimerism: interaction of grafts within a host? Blood 2010; 116:2706–12.
19. O'Donoghue K, Chan J, de la Fuente J, et al. Microchimerism in female bone marrow and bone decades after fetal mesenchymal stem-cell trafficking in pregnancy. Lancet 2004;364:179–82.
20. Raghupathy R, Al Mutawa E, Makhseed M, et al. Modulation of cytokine production by dydrogesterone in lymphocytes from women with recurrent miscarriage. BJOG 2005;112:1096–101.
21. von Wolff M, Thaler CJ, Strowitzki T, et al. Regulated expression of cytokines in human endometrium throughout the menstrual cycle: dysregulation in habitual abortion. Mol Hum Reprod 2000;6:627–34.

22. Schumacher A, Brachwitz N, Sohr S, et al. Human chorionic gonadotrophin attracts regulatory T cells into the fetal-maternal interface during human pregnancy. J Immunol 2009;182:5488–97.
23. Piosek ZM, Goegebeur Y, Klitlou L, et al. Plasma TNF-α levels are higher in early pregnancy in patients with secondary compared with primary recurrent miscarriage. Am J Reprod Immunol 2013;70:347–58.
24. Calleja-Agius J, Jauniaux E, Pizzey AR, et al. Investigation of systemic inflammatory response in first trimester pregnancy failure. Hum Reprod 2012;27:349–57.
25. Quack KC, Vassiliadou N, Pudney J, et al. Leukocyte activation in the decidua of chromosomally normal and abnormal fetuses from women with recurrent abortion. Hum Reprod 2001;16:949–55.
26. Bradford-Hill A. The environment and disease: association or causation? Proc R Soc Med 1965;9:295–300.
27. Lund M, Nielsen HS, Hviid TV, et al. Hereditary thrombophilia and recurrent pregnancy loss: a cohort study of pregnancy outcome and obstetric complications. Hum Reprod 2010;25:2978–84.
28. Jablonowska B, Selbing A, Palfi M, et al. Prevention of recurrent spontaneous abortion by intravenous immunoglobulin: a double-blind placebo-controlled trial. Hum Reprod 1999;14:838–41.
29. Christiansen OB, Pedersen B, Rosgaard A, et al. A randomized, double-blind, placebo-controlled trial of intravenous immunoglobulin in the prevention of recurrent miscarriage: evidence for a therapeutic effect in women with secondary recurrent miscarriage. Hum Reprod 2002;17:809–16.
30. Brigham SA, Conlon C, Farquharson RG. A longitudinal study of pregnancy outcome following idiopathic recurrent miscarriage. Hum Reprod 1999;14:2868–71.
31. Munné S, Chen S, Fischer J, et al. Preimplantation genetic diagnosis reduces pregnancy loss in women aged 35 years and older with a history of recurrent miscarriage. Fertil Steril 2005;84:331–5.
32. Glueck CJ, Wang P, Goldenberg N, et al. Pregnancy outcomes among women with polycystic ovary syndrome treated with metformin. Hum Reprod 2002;17:2858–64.
33. Yudkin PL, Stratton IM. How to deal with regression to the mean in intervention studies. Lancet 1996;347:241–3.
34. Christiansen OB. Transabdominal cervicoisthmic cerclage in the management of recurrent second trimester miscarriage and preterm delivery. BJOG 1996;103:595–6.
35. Stray-Pedersen B, Stray-Pedersen S. Etiological factors and subsequent reproductive performance in 195 couples with a history of habitual abortion. Am J Obstet Gynecol 1984;148:140–6.
36. Kutteh WH. Antiphospholipid antibody-associated recurrent pregnancy loss: treatment with heparin and low-dose aspirin is superior to low-dose aspirin alone. Am J Obstet Gynecol 1996;174:1584–9.
37. Rai R, Cohen H, Dave M, et al. Randomised controlled trial of aspirin and aspirin plus heparin in pregnant women with recurrent miscarriage associated with phospholipid antibodies (or antiphospholipid antibodies). BMJ 1997;314:253–7.
38. Kaandorp SP, Goddijn M, van der Post JAM. Aspirin plus heparin or aspirin alone in women with recurrent miscarriage. N Engl J Med 2010;362:1586–96.
39. The German RSA/IVIV Group. Intravenous immunoglobulin in the prevention of recurrent miscarriage. BJOG 1994;101:1072–7.

40. Stern J, Coulam CB. Mechanism of recurrent spontaneous abortion. I. Ultrasonographic findings. Am J Obstet Gynecol 1992;166:1844–52.
41. Ober C, Karrison T, Odem RR, et al. Mononuclear-cell immunisation in prevention of recurrent miscarriages: a randomised trial. Lancet 1999;354:365–9.
42. Stephenson MD, Kutteh WH, Purkiss S, et al. Intravenous immunoglobulin and idiopathic secondary recurrent miscarriage: a multicentered randomized placebo-controlled trial. Hum Reprod 2010;25:2203–9.
43. Brenner B, Hoffman R, Blumenfeld Z, et al. Gestational outcome in thrombophilic women with recurrent pregnancy loss treated with enoxaparin. Thromb Haemost 2000;83:693–7.
44. Grandone E, Brancaccio V, Colaizzo D, et al. Preventing adverse obstetric outcomes in women with genetic thrombophilia. Fertil Steril 2002;78:371–5.
45. Thompson SG, Higgins JPT. Can meta-analysis help target interventions at individuals most likely to benefit? Lancet 2005;365:341–6.
46. Hutton B, Sharma R, Fergusson D, et al. Use of intravenous immunoglobulin for treatment of recurrent miscarriage: a systematic review. BJOG 2007;114: 134–42.
47. Ata B, Tan SL, Shehata F, et al. A systematic review of intravenous immunoglobulin for treatment of unexplained recurrent miscarriage. Fertil Steril 2011;95: 1080–5.
48. Christiansen OB, Mathiesen O, Husth M. Placebo-controlled trial of treatment of unexplained secondary recurrent spontaneous abortions and recurrent late spontaneous abortions with i.v. immunoglobulin. Hum Reprod 1995;10:2690–5.
49. Christiansen OB, Larsen EC, Husth M, et al. Intravenous immunoglobulin and recurrent miscarriage. Fertil Steril 2011;7:e35.
50. Myakis S, Lockshin MD, Atsuma T, et al. International consensus statement on an update on the update of the classification criteria for the definite antiphospholipid syndrome (APS). J Thromb Haemost 2006;4:295–306.
51. Mueller-Eckhardt G, Mallmann P, Neppert J, et al. Immunogenetic and serological investigations in nonpregnant and in pregnant women with a history of recurrent spontaneous abortions. J Reprod Immunol 1994;27:95–109.
52. Clark DA. Intravenous immunoglobulin and idiopathic secondary recurrent miscarriage: methodological problems. Hum Reprod 2011;26:2586–91.

The Evolving Role of Genetics in Reproductive Medicine

Paul R. Brezina, MD, MBA[a,b,c,*], William G. Kearns, PhD[d,e]

KEYWORDS

- Genetics • Reproductive • Preimplantation genetic screening
- Preimplantation genetic diagnosis • Preimplantation • Chorionic villus sampling
- Amniocentesis • Cell-free DNA

KEY POINTS

- Genetics is increasingly being applied to reproductive medicine for both diagnosis and treatment.
- Preconception genetic testing, including testing for carrier states of conditions such as cystic fibrosis and hemoglobinopathies, will be increasingly used. There is an increasing trend to de-emphasize race to determine the appropriate testing.
- Antenatal genetic testing includes time-tested diagnostic evaluations such as chorionic villus sampling and amniocentesis. In addition, newer minimally invasive testing modalities are currently being developed and applied. The application of these tests is likely to increase in the future.
- Preimplantation genetic testing, including testing for specific genetic diseases and aneuploidy, is the practice of analyzing a biopsied sample of an egg or embryo obtained through in vitro fertilization. The ever improving accuracy and growing applications associated with this technology will likely lead to increased utilization.

Continued

Pertinent Disclosures and Conflicts of Interest: None.

Sources of Funding: None.

Contributors: P.R. Brezina primarily searched the literature. P.R. Brezina wrote the first draft of the article; W.G. Kearns edited the article and M.A. Kutteh advised on the content of the article, assisted in the literature search, and contributed to the writing of the article. P.R. Brezina is guarantor.

[a] Reproductive Endocrinology and Infertility, Fertility Associates of Memphis, 80 Humphreys Center, Suite 307, Memphis, TN 38120, USA; [b] Department of Obstetrics and Gynecology, Vanderbilt University Medical Center, B-1100 Medical Center North, Nashville, TN 37232, USA; [c] Department of Surgery, MS133, Room B3019, St. Jude Children's Research Hospital, 262 Danny Thomas Place, Memphis, TN 38105-3678, USA; [d] Department of Gynecology and Obstetrics, Johns Hopkins Medical Institutions, Phipps 264, 600 North Wolfe Street, Baltimore, MD 21287, USA; [e] Preimplantation Genetics, The Center for Preimplantation Genetics, Lab-Corp, 15001 Shady Grove Road, Suite 200, Rockville, MD 20850, USA

* Corresponding author. Reproductive Endocrinology and Infertility, Fertility Associates of Memphis, 80 Humphreys Center, Suite 307, Memphis, TN 38120, USA.

E-mail address: pbrezina@fertilitymemphis.com

Obstet Gynecol Clin N Am 41 (2014) 41–55

http://dx.doi.org/10.1016/j.ogc.2013.10.006

obgyn.theclinics.com

0889-8545/14/$ – see front matter © 2014 Elsevier Inc. All rights reserved.

Continued

- Genetic analysis following fetal demise is now capable of evaluating the genetic karyotype of products of conception without growth in culture, through microarray technology. In addition, certain microarray evaluations are capable of ruling out maternal cell contamination. These advances may improve the diagnosis and future treatment of women suffering from failed pregnancy.
- It is incumbent on clinicians, however, to ensure that these interventions are used in a responsible, equitable, and ethical manner.

INTRODUCTION

At its core, reproductive medicine attempts to explain how human life is created and how it develops throughout pregnancy. Based on this understanding, therapies are developed and used to maximize outcomes. Specifically, increased pregnancy rates, decreased incidence of obstetric complications and miscarriage, and the avoidance of fetuses affected by birth defects or other deficiencies are the stated goal of much of the current research in reproductive medicine. The role of genetic testing to guide medical decision making in this regard is sizable and will likely continue to grow in the future.

Genetic evaluations within reproductive medicine may be subdivided into 4 main categories:

1. Preconception genetic testing: The genetic evaluation of prospective parents before pregnancy
2. Antenatal genetic testing: The genetic evaluation of women who are currently pregnant to determine the genetic makeup of the developing fetus
3. Preimplantation genetic testing: The genetic evaluation of an embryo, before uterine transfer, via an embryo biopsy during an in vitro fertilization (IVF) procedure
4. Genetic analysis following fetal demise: The genetic evaluation of the products of conception following a failed pregnancy

This article outlines each of these broad categories and describes the current appropriate applications of these technologies.

PRECONCEPTION GENETIC TESTING

Preconception genetic testing is the genetic evaluation of prospective parents before pregnancy (**Box 1**). Many individuals have a specific family history of certain genetic disorders, but many may also be at risk for unknown genetic diseases. Preconception genetic testing can be based on a couple's ethnicity or the medical history of a genetic

---

Box 1
Preconception genetic testing

- Many individuals may be unknown carriers of certain genetic diseases
- Preconception testing for a variety of genetic diseases is increasingly recommended in phenotypically normal individuals
- Technological advances have improved the accuracy and have decreased the cost of such testing
- Race is increasingly de-emphasized to determine appropriate testing panels

disease segregating in their families. Most genetic diseases identified because of ethnicity are autosomal recessive disorders (AR), and require 2 mutations to have the disease. For a fetus to be affected with an AR disorder, each parent must pass along a mutation and, therefore, the fetal risk is 25%. One example of an AR disorder is cystic fibrosis (CF). In fact the carrier rate for CF among all individuals in the United States is 1 in 37, but may be as high as 1 in 27 in certain ethnic groups.[1]

Genetic diseases segregating in a patient's family can be autosomal dominant (AD), AR, or X-linked (XL). For AD disorders, if the fetus has the mutation the baby will have the disease. An example of an AD disorder is Huntington disease. XL disorders exist on the X chromosome, and can be XL dominant or XL recessive. In simplistic terms, most XL disorders are caused by unaffected carrier mothers passing along their mutant X-chromosome to their affected sons. An example of an XL disorder is fragile X.

Various modalities and technologies are used for preconception genetic testing, and these test for the most common, though not necessarily all, mutations associated with the genetic disease. Most testing technologies include direct mutation analysis by genotyping, duplication/deletion analysis, and DNA sequencing, and can use classic linkage analysis.

Preconception genetic testing for couples considering pregnancy specifically to determine the carrier status for certain genetic AR disorders has been available for some time.[2] The list of recommended AR inherited disorders to evaluate in the context of preconception evaluation is limited and is primarily based on the recommendations of 2 societies.[3,4] In addition, these societies often differ in exactly which tests are recommended.

Common conditions currently tested in a preconception genetic evaluation based on ethnicity include hemoglobinopathies (sickle cell trait, C trait, thalassemia trait, hemoglobin E), CF, Tay-Sachs disease, Canavan disease, familial dysautonomia, mucolipidosis IV, Niemann-Pick disease type A, Fanconi anemia group C, Bloom syndrome, Gaucher disease, and spinal muscular atrophy.

In the past, most preconception genetic testing was tailored to patients according to their ethnic background, as the carrier rate for specific disorders is known to differ among various ethnic groups. As the population of pan-ethnic societies, such as the United States, continues to become increasingly interracial, such targeted testing is becoming increasingly problematic.[3,4] A recent bulletin by the American Congress of Obstetrics and Gynecology (ACOG) recently noted when evaluating this subject that "it is becoming increasingly difficult to assign a single ethnicity to individuals."[3,4] Consequently, many experts now recommend offering universal carrier genetic testing for many of these AR disorders within the context of preconception counseling to all patients, regardless of their ethnic background.

When a positive result is obtained for a genetic disorder, the specifics of this result and its clinical risk must be explained clearly to the patient either by their clinician or a genetic counselor. In addition, patients should be counseled on available strategies to minimize the risk of having an affected child, including preimplantation genetic diagnosis within the context of an IVF cycle. Referral to a reproductive endocrinologist or geneticist familiar with these technologies may be advised.

ANTENATAL GENETIC TESTING

A central focus of obstetric care for many years has been to identify fetal disorders during pregnancy. In the age of elective terminations following the *Roe v. Wade* United Sates Supreme Court decision (410 U.S. 113; 1973), information regarding the status of the developing fetus has been used to guide medical decisions. In general, the baseline incidence of some type of birth defect is approximately 3%.[5] For many of these defects, detailed ultrasonography and other methods are used to identify specific anatomic anomalies. However, in most instances these anomalies are associated with a euploid (normal) genetic complement (either 46,XX or 46,XY). Although there may also be specific genetic abnormalities associated with this myriad of birth defects in euploid fetuses, genetic evaluation is currently not the modality used to identify such problems. Therefore, the remainder of the discussion in this article focuses on the genetic evaluations used to identify aneuploid (abnormal) genetic complements in the developing fetus during pregnancy.

The Basics of Aneuploidy

Chromosomal aneuploidy, a condition in which either too many or too few chromosomes are present on any 1 of the 23 chromosome pairs, is a common occurrence in human reproduction (**Box 2**). During the process, ovulation and fertilization human oocytes (eggs) and sperm undergo a series of organized genetic separation events known as meiosis. A simplified view of one of these events is outlined in **Fig. 1**. In this scheme, a diploid (2 copies of a chromosome) is divided into 2; 1 represents an ovulated egg and the other a discarded polar body. This haploid (having one copy of each chromosome) egg then is fertilized by another haploid sperm, producing a diploid embryo having 2 copies of each chromosome, one from each parent. In reality, however, this is a very simplified and incomplete summary of this process. Maternal meiosis in fact includes 2 phases of meiosis.

This process of meiosis is complex. If there is an uneven split of the chromosome pairs during meiosis, as is shown in **Fig. 2**, the resulting egg either has 2 or no copies of the chromosome. Following fertilization with sperm, this may result in either an extra copy of a chromosome (trisomy) or only 1 copy, not 2 copies, of a chromosome (monosomy). There are 23 chromosome pairs, and a splitting error on any 1 of these chromosomes results in a chromosomal complement that is unbalanced and generally not compatible with life. In fact, the only aneuploidy errors that can be compatible with a live birth are errors in the number of sex chromosomes (eg, 45X, 47XXY, 47XYY) and trisomy in chromosomes 13, 18, or 21. Of these trisomies, chromosome 21 (Down syndrome) is generally associated with fetal survival past 1 year of age, and is associated with a host of developmental and health problems.

The focus of fetal genetic testing has traditionally focused on identifying trisomies in 13, 18, or 21 or X-chromosome monosomy, because these errors are the only problems that could be associated with a live birth. Aneuploidy errors on other chromosomes, while common, generally result in a failed pregnancy early in the first trimester before traditional testing (such as sampling of chorionic villi or amniocentesis) can practically be performed. However, technologies are currently available

---

Box 2
Antenatal genetic testing

- Aneuploidy is common in human embryos

- Modalities for testing the genetic status of the human fetus in utero have existed for some time, and include chorionic villus sampling and amniocentesis

- Evaluation of maternal cell-free DNA is a minimally invasive testing modality that offers the ability to identify aneuploidy in many cases. The application of this test is likely to increase in the future

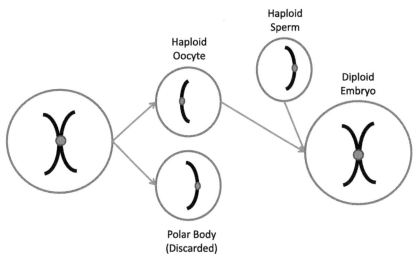

Fig. 1. Normal chromosomal division. This scheme depicts a normal meiotic division of one chromosome in which a diploid chromosome divides into haploid copies. One of these haploid copies joins with a haploid sperm, resulting in a diploid embryo.

that permit a more complete and, in some cases, less invasive fetal genetic evaluation. The following summarizes some of these interventions.

Chorionic Villus Sampling and Amniocentesis

Chorionic villus sampling (CVS) and amniocentesis are technologies that have been used for decades to determine whether aneuploidy or structural chromosome aberrations are present in the developing fetus. Often, these interventions are used after

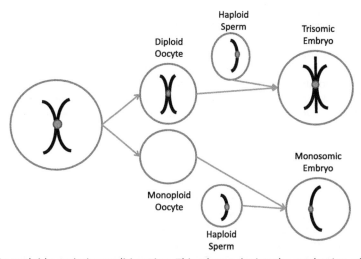

Fig. 2. Aneuploidy: meiotic nondisjunction. This scheme depicts the mechanism of meiotic nondisjunction whereby a diploid chromosome fails to divide into 2 haploid copies. After joining with a haploid sperm, this results in an embryo that has either 3 chromosomal copies (trisomy) or 1 chromosomal copy (monosomy).

there is some abnormality detected on ultrasonography or certain types of blood tests (hat screen for maternal proteins) commonly performed to determine the risk of aneuploidy in early pregnancy. In addition, women of advanced maternal age (>35 years) are often offered either CVS or amniocentesis. Both CVS and amniocentesis work by surgically obtaining and genetically evaluating fetal cells. In CVS, these cells are obtained by sampling chorionic villi via ultrasound-guided needle biopsy between 10 and 14 weeks of gestation.[6] Amniocentesis is performed by needle aspiration of amniotic fluid around 15 weeks of gestation.[6] At present, the samples obtained by either CVS or amniocentesis may be evaluated to generate a fetal karyotype or other targeted single-gene genetic testing as dictated by the clinical context.

However, CVS and amniocentesis have certain risks. First, the procedure of invasive sampling used with both these approaches is associated with pregnancy loss. The rate of pregnancy loss is estimated to be less than 1%, but is certainly not 0%.[6] In addition, there is some level of maternal physical discomfort and stress associated with the performance of these procedures. Furthermore, CVS may provide spurious results in patients with a condition known as confined placental mosaicism, a condition whereby the placenta possesses a mixture of aneuploid and euploid cells while the fetus is euploid.

Cell-Free Fetal DNA Evaluation

It has been documented that nucleated cells derived from the fetal-placental unit can be detected circulating in maternal blood at a level of 1 to 6 cells per milliliter of maternal blood.[7,8] More commonly observed in the maternal blood circulation are cellular fragments of DNA, generally thought to be placental in origin. These placentally derived DNA fragments actually comprise approximately 3% to 6% of all circulating cell-free DNA in maternal plasma.[5,9,10] These fragments may be detected very early in pregnancy, but are not reliably present until later in the first trimester.[7,8]

In 2007, Down syndrome (trisomy 21) was detected by genetic evaluation of these DNA fragments isolated from maternal blood.[11] Since this landmark case, the utilization of cell-free fetal DNA evaluation has become increasingly common. At present there are commercially available platforms that evaluate trisomies for chromosomes 13, 18, and 21 using this technique. However, these testing modalities are still considered a screen, and a diagnostic follow-up by CVS or amniocentesis is recommended.

Unlike CVS or amniocentesis, cell-free fetal DNA evaluation is noninvasive and is not associated with any rate of pregnancy loss resulting from the performance of the procedure. In addition, the test may be performed very early in pregnancy at approximately 10 weeks' gestation, well before when CVS or amniocentesis is possible. As this technology evolves and supportive data accumulate, an increased diagnostic role for this technology may be appropriate.

PREIMPLANTATION GENETIC TESTING

An IVF cycle consists of administering injectable gonadotropins to women and inducing controlled ovarian hyperstimulation whereby more than the usual number of ovarian follicles are recruited and matured.[12,13] The oocytes within these follicles are then surgically harvested and inseminated with sperm. Typically resultant embryos are then grown in vitro until either 3 or 5 days of development, at which time the 1 or 2 best embryos are placed into the uterus and the remaining embryos are cryopreserved. It is possible to biopsy a cell(s) from developing embryos before embryo transfer, and to perform various genetic analyses that determine which embryos would be optimal for either embryo transfer or cryopreservation. Therefore, the purpose of preimplantation genetic testing is to improve the likelihood of carrying a pregnancy to term and giving birth to a healthy baby.

When first introduced around 1990, preimplantation genetic testing was used exclusively to determine whether embryos harbored a specific genetic mutation that was known to exist from parental DNA analysis.[14–16] This practice of evaluating embryos for a known parental genetic defect is known as preimplantation genetic diagnosis (PGD). As aneuploidy is the most significant reason for pregnancy failure, the technology of evaluating biopsied cells from embryos was then used to determine the ploidy status of embryos before uterine transfer.[17,18] This evaluation of embryonic cells for aneuploidy from healthy parents, rather than a single genetic defect, is termed preimplantation genetic screening (PGS). PGD or PGS may be helpful to those who have experienced problems with infertility, recurrent pregnancy loss (miscarriages), or unsuccessful IVF cycles. PGD may also be useful to couples who are at risk for passing an inherited genetic condition on to their children (**Box 3**).

Preimplantation Genetic Diagnosis

As already discussed, PGD is the practice of evaluating embryos for a known parental genetic defect. The utilization of this technology is now widely accepted as appropriate in couples harboring a known genetic abnormality.[13] The chief uses of PGD are outlined here.

Single-gene disorders

PGD for single-gene mutations diagnoses specific genetic mutations that are documented in the parents and segregating within their extended family. This goal is accomplished using polymerase chain reaction (PCR) to amplify the DNA of the chromosome where the gene of interest resides.[19] DNA sequencing then identifies the specific gene

---

Box 3
Preimplantation genetic testing (PGT)

- PGT is achieved by obtaining a cellular biopsy from a developing human oocyte or embryo obtained via an in vitro fertilization cycle, evaluating the genetic composition of this sample, and using information gained from this process to determine optimal embryos for subsequent uterine transfer.
- PGT is performed by:
  - Obtaining cell(s) from either a developing embryo or oocyte
  - Genetic analysis of cells obtained at biopsy
- PGT is subdivided into 2 broad categories
  - Preimplantation genetic diagnosis (PGD)
    - The purpose of PGD is to prevent the birth of affected children from parents with a known genetic abnormality
    - PGD is widely acknowledged as acceptable for routine clinical application
  - Preimplantation genetic screening (PGS)
    - Attempts to identify aneuploidy in embryos to improve pregnancy success in certain patient populations
    - Parents with no identified genetic defect or disease
    - PGS remains controversial for routine application
- The results obtained by PGT may not always reflect the fetus' genetic composition.

mutation, and linkage analysis identifies surrounding markers used to determine recombination and whether the DNA of the sperm and oocyte is amplified.[20,21]

Structural chromosome aberrations

In couples with recurrent pregnancy loss (RPL) and/or a documented balanced reciprocal/Robertsonian translocation (**Fig. 3**) or chromosomal inversion in one or both parents, PGD coupled with IVF has been shown to have some benefit in improving pregnancy and live birth rates.[22–24] Fluorescence in situ hybridization (FISH) has traditionally been used to identify the presence of translocation imbalances in PGD translocation cases. FISH identifies chromosomal balances or imbalances, but is unable to rule out the presence of a balanced translocation chromosome. However over recent years microarrays have been increasingly utilized. Microarrays are able to simultaneously identify genetic imbalances caused by the parental translocation or inversion chromosome, and evaluate all 23 pairs of chromosomes from a single cell or cells. As with FISH, microarrays can only identify genetic balances or imbalances, and cannot differentiate the presence of a translocation chromosome from its normal counterpart.[23,25]

Because of the complexities of PGD, all patients must be adequately counseled on the risks and limitations of PGD, preferably with the aid of a specialized physician, geneticist, or genetic counselor. Furthermore, antenatal genetic testing is still recommended in all patients undergoing PGS.[13]

Preimplantation Genetic Screening

PGS determines whether aneuploidy exists for any of the 23 pairs of chromosomes. The transfer of euploid embryos seems to play a significant role in implantation and fetal development. Determining which embryos are best has been a subject of much debate since the advent of IVF technology in the late 1970s. Traditionally the use of morphology (the visual appearance of embryos) has been the principal modality of choosing optimal embryos for uterine transfer.[26] However, the implantation rate per transferred embryo in most clinics rarely exceeds 40%.[27] Therefore, many investigators have for some time been searching to establish other diagnostic methods that are

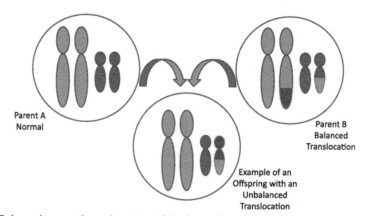

Fig. 3. Balanced parental translocations. This scheme depicts the mechanism by which parents who harbor a balanced chromosomal translocation may have offspring with unbalanced translocation errors. Of note, parents harboring balanced chromosomal translocations may also have offspring with different chromosomal combinations that may be phenotypically or genetically normal.

capable of determining embryo quality more accurately than morphology alone. PGS improves the implantation rate and delivery rate for RPL patients and, possibly, other clinical indications.

PGS, unlike PGD, has been and continues to be a controversial technology. Recent studies indicate that approximately more than 70% of all first-trimester miscarriages are the result of chromosomal aneuploidy.[13] Because so many early miscarriages are due to aneuploidy, PGS seems to be a reasonable intervention to improve the efficiency with which euploid (chromosomally normal) embryos are selected for uterine transfer in IVF cycles. Classic studies have reported that first-trimester miscarriages resulting from aneuploidy are disproportionately concentrated on select chromosomes.[28,29] These data are based on karyotype analysis of failed pregnancies that developed far enough to have tissue available for genetic analysis.[28,29] Consequently, clinics performing PGS in the early days of the technology focused on detecting aneuploidy on only select chromosomes using FISH, which typically evaluates between 5 and 14 chromosome pairs rather than all 23 chromosome pairs.[30,31] Traditionally, the PGS biopsy was exclusively performed at approximately 3 days of embryonic development following fertilization.[30,31] Unfortunately, this approach failed to lead to improvements in clinical pregnancy rates, and this lack of efficacy was widely referenced following a landmark article by Mastenbroek and colleagues[32] in the *New England Journal of Medicine*. Subsequently, similar articles cast further doubt on the benefits of PGS, and position statements from major medical societies formally discouraged its use.[16,33,34]

Further research, however, elucidated several biological limitations that could explain the prior shortcomings of clinically applied PGS. First, studies have repeatedly documented that embryos at day 3 of development have high levels of mosaicism.[35,36] A photograph of an embryo undergoing a day-3 biopsy is shown in **Fig. 4**. Mosaicism is a condition whereby a single developing embryo comprises more than 1 distinct genetic cell line. In other words, mosaic embryos may have euploid (normal) and aneuploid (abnormal) cell lines within a single embryo. Studies evaluating this phenomenon have concluded that as many as 50% of all embryos may be mosaic at day 3 of development.[35,36] Consequently, a biopsy performed at day 3 of development may produce a result that is not representative of the entire embryo.[13] It is clear that embryos developmentally change during differentiation to the blastocyst stage of development. Data have shown that mosaicism is greatly reduced in blastocysts, to approximately 5%.[13,37]

Another limitation of traditionally performed PGS was the use of FISH for determination of chromosomal aneuploidies. FISH typically evaluates between 5 and 14 rather than all 23 chromosome pairs.[38] Recent studies have indicated that embryonic

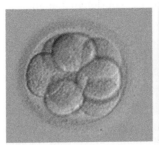 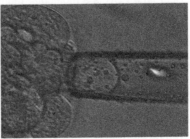

Fig. 4. Cleavage-stage embryo. These photographs show an embryo at the cleavage stage. On the right is a photograph of a cleavage-stage biopsy.

aneuploidy occurs in clinically significant amounts in all 23 chromosome pairs.[39] Therefore, FISH is incapable of diagnosing many of the chromosomal abnormalities commonly found in developing embryos.

Realization of these 2 principal limitations have led many genetic laboratories to offer PGS using technologies evaluating the chromosomal status of all 23 chromosome pairs on cells obtained from differentiating blastocysts, typically reached by day 5 or day 6 of embryo development. A photograph of an embryo undergoing a day-5 biopsy is shown in **Fig. 5**. The clinical pregnancy rates using this approach have been reported to be markedly superior to the traditional approach of performing PGS.[40,41] For example, a recent study evaluating more than 4500 embryos using determination of 23 chromosome pairs found clinical pregnancy rates in women suffering from RPL to be significantly improved in comparison with similar studies using FISH PGS.[40] In addition, pregnancy rates were further improved when 23-chromosome-pair evaluation PGS was performed on blastocyst stage embryos (day 5/6 of development), compared with when the biopsy was performed on embryos at day 3 of development.[30,40,42] Similar results have been reported consistently by many clinics in the United States and around the world.[30,42,43] This trend has led to a renewed interest in PGS, although it still remains to be determined whether PGS is an efficacious technology and which patient populations are best served by PGS.

Evaluation technologies using all 23 chromosome pairs are complex and differ in their experimental approach. The 2 most common technologies are microarrays and real-time PCR.[13] Both of these technologies rely on obtaining embryonic DNA, amplifying this DNA, and evaluating the amplified product using microarrays or real-time PCR. This amplification process is a potential source of error, as failure to amplify the entire embryonic DNA genome could produce a false result. In addition, all amplification protocols must be performed under sterile conditions so as to avoid any exogenous contamination.

There are 2 types of microarrays, single-nucleotide polymorphism (SNP) and comparative genomic hybridization (CGH). SNP arrays directly evaluate ploidy by genotyping alleles on a dense chip of approximately 300,000 genetic markers.[13] CGH arrays, by contrast, evaluate far fewer genetic markers and determine ploidy by comparing the clinical DNA sample with male and female reference DNA samples.[13] Each of these microarray platforms have advantages and disadvantages. SNP arrays can identify loss of heterozygosity, consanguinity, and uniparental disomy whereas CGH arrays cannot, because of their ratio labeling protocol.

Significant advantages of CGH arrays are that that they may be performed in 12 hours and provide the IVF clinic the opportunity to transfer the embryos on day 6 of embryo development, potentially eliminate the need for an embryo freeze and a frozen embryo transfer, and can determine large clinically significant deletions or duplications. Real-time PCR is a molecular technique that determines the presence or

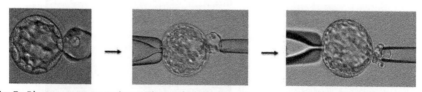

Fig. 5. Blastocyst-stage embryo. These photographs show an embryo at the blastocyst stage. The leftmost photo shows the herniation of trophectoderm (TE) cells after the application of a laser to breach the zona pellucida. The next 2 photographs show the process of obtaining a sheet of TE cells that will be analyzed for preimplantation genetic screening.

absence of 3 to 5 chromosomal loci on the test sample DNA. It then quantitatively compares the chromosome copy number with a reference DNA sample. Real-time PCR can reliably determine aneuploidy in approximately 6 hours and can also provide IVF clinics the ability to transfer embryos on day 6 of development. One disadvantage of real-time PCR is the inability to determine structural chromosome aberrations.

Evidence for the Clinical Application of PGS

Studies from centers using PGS on day-5 and day-6 blastocysts show promising results, with transferred embryos generating pregnancy rates greater than 72%.[30,40,42] However, a central criticism of the widespread use of PGS is a lack of randomized controlled trials that conclusively show the procedure to be beneficial. While some prospective trials currently do exist that support the application of PGS to improve pregnancy outcome, further studies are required before PGS will be more broadly accepted.[13,43,44]

Despite the lack of support from professional societies and the lack of large, randomized controlled trials definitively demonstrating the benefits of the technology, PGS comprises the major part of all preimplantation genetic testing internationally, and is being increasingly used.[45] However, the patient population for which PGS may be appropriate is unclear at present.[13] Many PGS clinics have traditionally recommended PGS for couples with risk factors believed to be associated with embryonic aneuploidy such as unexplained RPL, severe male factor, and advanced maternal age. However, in recent years many clinics have liberally expanded the use of PGS to many women without such risk factors. In fact, some clinics broadly recommend PGS to virtually all IVF patients as a strategy to improve pregnancy rates in all couples battling infertility. The debate surrounding the appropriate patient populations for PGS is currently in flux, and will likely be a source of debate for years to come.

Limitations of PGS

Despite the positive data emerging within the field of PGS, there are tangible technical and biological limitations to the technology. The limitations of FISH PGS evaluation and the use of biopsy taken from day-3 embryos are significant, as discussed earlier. In addition, technical limitations surrounding the use of both SNP and CGH arrays and real-time PCR may produce spurious results if not properly validated and experimentally performed.[13]

Perhaps the most significant source of error from PGS using 23-chromosome-pair evaluation on cleavage stage (day 3) or blastocysts (day 5/6 of development) is the presence of mosaicism within the developing embryo. Clearly it is not possible to perform genetic testing on every cell of an embryo, as this is not compatible with having a viable embryo available for uterine transfer. The best recommendation is to perform 23-chromosome-pair PGS on blastocysts.

The aforementioned limitations of PGS demand that patients be adequately counseled on its risks and limitations, preferably with the aid of a specialized physician, geneticist, or genetic counselor. Furthermore, antenatal genetic testing is still recommended in all patients undergoing PGS.[13]

New technologies associated with PGS are producing data suggesting that the procedure could be a valuable adjunct to assisted reproductive technologies in the future, to enhance pregnancy success in most patients. Defining the exact benefit conferred by PGS and determining exactly which patient populations could be best served by it, however, is currently controversial. In the near future, the field should commission large and high-quality studies that will attempt to answer these questions. Despite this lack of definitive data, however, PGS is increasingly being

---

Box 4
Genetic analysis following fetal demise

- Aneuploidy is extremely common in embryogenesis and is responsible for the lion's share of pregnancy losses in the early first trimester
- Genetic analysis following fetal demise is now capable of evaluating the genetic karyotype of products of conception without growth in culture through microarray technology
- Certain microarray evaluations are capable of ruling out maternal cell contamination
- These advances may improve diagnosis and future treatment of women suffering from failed pregnancy

---

applied to patients with ever expanding clinical indications. Although there are few large, randomized controlled studies defining the benefits of PGS, clinical data emerging from many PGS laboratories around the world are encouraging. Therefore, the judicious use of PGS seems reasonable at present, as the preponderance of available current evidence suggests that some couples may derive benefit from this technology. Only with time will the role of PGS be clearly defined.

GENETIC ANALYSIS FOLLOWING FETAL DEMISE

As discussed earlier in the PGS section, chromosomal aneuploidy is extremely common in embryogenesis and is responsible for the lion's share of pregnancy losses in the early first trimester. However, determining whether aneuploidy existed in early first trimester losses has traditionally been difficult by routine karyotypic analysis, which requires the culture of cells followed by the generation of a G-banded karyotype. Failed cultures attributable to the presence of toxic substances and/or toxic cell products prohibit cell synchronization required for G-banding of metaphase chromosomes. Another important issue of routine karyotypic analysis of products of conception (POC) tissue is maternal cell contamination. Because of maternal cell contamination, with a 46,XX G-banded karyotype one cannot be certain that the analyzed cells are fetal or maternal in origin, and are therefore of little clinical value.

The introduction of SNP microarrays has dramatically changed the way first-trimester pregnancy losses are being evaluated. Arrays are capable of amplifying DNA samples from POC cells without requiring cell culture, thus permitting the analysis of small initial samples without the requirement of metaphase chromosome synchronization. Furthermore, SNP arrays determine genotypes, and if a maternal DNA sample is run with the POC tissue, one can differentiate a fetal 46,XX karyotype from a maternal 46,XX karyotype. Through these improvements, evaluation of first-trimester POCs through SNP microarrays has become an important component of the evaluation of RPL (**Box 4**).

SUMMARY

The past several decades have witnessed a dramatic increase in genetic diagnostics and therapeutic interventions offered to patients. Reproductive medicine is no exception to this statement. As our understanding of genetics and its relation to disease expands, there surely will be an ever expanding role for genetics within reproductive medicine. It is incumbent on clinicians, however, to ensure that these interventions are used in a responsible, equitable, and ethical manner.

ACKNOWLEDGMENTS

The authors thank Drs William Kutteh and Raymond Ke for their help in writing this article. They also extend gratitude to Michael A. Kutteh for his assistance in the preparation and submission of this article. His contributions are greatly appreciated, as he helped to facilitate the timely submission of this article.

REFERENCES

1. Strom CM, Crossley B, Buller-Buerkle A, et al. Cystic fibrosis testing 8 years on: lessons learned from carrier screening and sequencing analysis. Genet Med 2011;13(2):166–72.
2. Pletcher BA, Bocian M, American College of Medical Genetics. Preconception and prenatal testing of biologic fathers for carrier status. American College of Medical Genetics. Genet Med 2006;8(2):134–5.
3. ACOG Committee on Genetics. ACOG Committee Opinion No. 442: preconception and prenatal carrier screening for genetic diseases in individuals of Eastern European Jewish descent. Obstet Gynecol 2009;114(4):950–3.
4. American College of Obstetricians and Gynecologists Committee on Genetics. ACOG Committee Opinion No. 486: update on carrier screening for cystic fibrosis. Obstet Gynecol 2011;117(4):1028–31.
5. Bodurtha J, Strauss JF 3rd. Genomics and perinatal care. N Engl J Med 2012; 366(1):64–73.
6. Simpson JL. Invasive procedures for prenatal diagnosis: any future left? Best Pract Res Clin Obstet Gynaecol 2012;26(5):625–38.
7. Go AT, van Vugt JM, Oudejans CB. Non-invasive aneuploidy detection using free fetal DNA and RNA in maternal plasma: recent progress and future possibilities. Hum Reprod Update 2011;17(3):372–82.
8. Ehrich M, Deciu C, Zwiefelhofer T, et al. Noninvasive detection of fetal trisomy 21 by sequencing of DNA in maternal blood: a study in a clinical setting. Am J Obstet Gynecol 2011;204(3):205.e1–11.
9. Chiu RW, Akolekar R, Zheng YW, et al. Non-invasive prenatal assessment of trisomy 21 by multiplexed maternal plasma DNA sequencing: large scale validity study. BMJ 2011;342:c7401. http://dx.doi.org/10.1136/bmj.c7401.
10. Rizzo JM, Buck MJ. Key principles and clinical applications of "next-generation" DNA sequencing. Cancer Prev Res (Phila) 2012;5:887–900.
11. Kido S, Sakuragi N, Bronner MP, et al. D21S418E identifies a cAMP-regulated gene located on chromosome 21q22.3 that is expressed in placental syncytiotrophoblast and choriocarcinoma cells. Genomics 1993; 17(1):256–9.
12. Brezina PR, Benner A, Rechitsky S, et al. Single-gene testing combined with single nucleotide polymorphism microarray preimplantation genetic diagnosis for aneuploidy: a novel approach in optimizing pregnancy outcome. Fertil Steril 2011;95:1786.
13. Brezina PR, Brezina DS, Kearns WG. Preimplantation genetic testing. BMJ 2012; 345:e5908.
14. ACOG Committee Opinion No. 430: preimplantation genetic screening for aneuploidy. Obstet Gynecol 2009;113(3):766–7.
15. Handyside A, Kontogianni EH, Hardy K, et al. Pregnancies from biopsied human preimplantation embryos sexed by Y-specific DNA amplification. Nature 1990; 344:768–70.

16. Practice Committee of Society for Assisted Reproductive Technology, Practice Committee of American Society for Reproductive Medicine. Preimplantation genetic testing: a Practice Committee opinion. Fertil Steril 2008;90:S136–43.
17. Hassold T, Chen N, Funkhouser J, et al. A cytogenetic study of 1000 spontaneous abortions. Ann Hum Genet 1980;44:151–78.
18. Menasha J, Levy B, Hirschhorn K, et al. Incidence and spectrum of chromosome abnormalities in spontaneous abortions: new insights from a 12-year study. Genet Med 2005;7:251–63.
19. Verlinsky Y, Cieslak J, Freidine M, et al. Pregnancies following preconception diagnosis of common aneuploidies by fluorescent in-situ hybridization. Hum Reprod 1995;10:1923–7.
20. Laurie AD, Hill AM, Harraway JR, et al. Preimplantation genetic diagnosis for hemophilia A using indirect linkage analysis and direct genotyping approaches. J Thromb Haemost 2010;8:783–9.
21. Cirulli ET, Goldstein DB. Uncovering the roles of rare variants in common disease through whole genome sequencing. Nat Rev Genet 2010;11:415–25.
22. Kuliev A, Verlinsky Y. Current features of preimplantation genetic diagnosis. Reprod Biomed Online 2002;5(3):294–9.
23. Treff NR, Northrop LE, Kasabwala K, et al. Single nucleotide polymorphism microarray-based concurrent screening of 24-chromosome aneuploidy and unbalanced translocations in preimplantation human embryos. Fertil Steril 2011; 95(5):1606–12.e2.
24. Otani T, Roche M, Mizuike M, et al. Preimplantation genetic diagnosis significantly improves the pregnancy outcome of translocation carriers with a history of recurrent miscarriage and unsuccessful pregnancies. Reprod Biomed Online 2006; 13(6):869–74.
25. Du L, Brezina PR, Benner AT, et al. The rate of de novo and inherited aneuploidy as determined by 23-chromosome single nucleotide polymorphism microarray (SNP) in embryos generated from parents with known chromosomal translocations. Fertil Steril 2011;96(3):S221.
26. Brezina PR, Zhao Y. The ethical, legal, and social issues impacted by modern assisted reproductive technologies. Obstet Gynecol Int 2012;2012:686253.
27. Ajduk A, Zernicka-Goetz M. Advances in embryo selection methods. F1000 Biol Rep 2012;4:11.
28. Monni G, Ibba RM, Zoppi MA. Prenatal genetic diagnosis through chorionic villus sampling. In: Milunsky A, Milunsky JM, editors. Genetic disorders and the fetus. 6th edition. Oxford (United Kingdom): Wiley-Blackwell; 2010.
29. Kearns WG, Pen R, Graham J, et al. Preimplantation genetic diagnosis and screening. Semin Reprod Med 2005;23(4):336–47.
30. Schoolcraft WB, Fragouli E, Stevens J, et al. Clinical application of comprehensive chromosomal screening at the blastocyst stage. Fertil Steril 2010;94: 1700–6.
31. Brezina PR, Kearns WG. Preimplantation genetic screening in the age of 23-chromosome evaluation; why FISH is no longer an acceptable technology. J Fertiliz In Vitro 2011;1:e103.
32. Mastenbroek S, Twisk M, Echten-Arends J, et al. In vitro fertilization with preimplantation genetic screening. N Engl J Med 2007;357:9–17.
33. Checa MA, Alonso-Coello P, Solà I, et al. IVF/ICSI with or without preimplantation genetic screening for aneuploidy in couples without genetic disorders: a systematic review and meta-analysis. J Assist Reprod Genet 2009;26: 273–83.

34. Mastenbroek S, Twisk M, van der Veen F, et al. Preimplantation genetic screening: a systematic review and meta-analysis of RCTs. Hum Reprod Update 2011;17: 454–66.
35. Harton GL, Magli MC, Lundin K, et al, European Society for Human Reproduction and Embryology (ESHRE), PGD Consortium/Embryology Special Interest Group. ESHRE PGD Consortium/Embryology Special Interest Group—best practice guidelines for polar body and embryo biopsy for preimplantation genetic diagnosis/screening (PGD/PGS). Hum Reprod 2011;26:41–6.
36. Munné S, Weier HU, Grifo J, et al. Chromosome mosaicism in human embryos. Biol Reprod 1994;51:373–9.
37. Brezina PR, Sun Y, Anchan RM, et al. Aneuploid embryos as determined by 23 single nucleotide polymorphism (SNP) microarray preimplantation genetic screening (PGS) possess the potential to genetically normalize during early development. Fertil Steril 2012;98(3):S108.
38. Harper JC, Sengupta SB. Preimplantation genetic diagnosis: state of the art 2011. Hum Genet 2012;131:175–86.
39. Brezina PR, Tobler K, Benner AT, et al. All 23 chromosomes have significant levels of aneuploidy in recurrent pregnancy loss couples. Fertil Steril 2012;97(3):S7.
40. Brezina PR, Tobler K, Benner AT, et al. In vitro fertilization (IVF) cycles and 4,873 embryos using 23-chromosome single nucleotide polymorphism (SNP) microarray preimplantation genetic screening (PGS). Fertil Steril 2012;97:S23–4.
41. Wells D, Alfarawati S, Fragouli E. Use of comprehensive chromosomal screening for embryo assessment: microarrays and CGH. Mol Hum Reprod 2008;14: 703–10.
42. Forman EJ, Tao X, Ferry KM, et al. Single embryo transfer with comprehensive chromosome screening results in improved ongoing pregnancy rates and decreased miscarriage rates. Hum Reprod 2012;27:1217–22.
43. Scott RT Jr, Upham KM, Forman EJ, et al. Blastocyst biopsy with comprehensive chromosome screening and fresh embryo transfer significantly increases in vitro fertilization implantation and delivery rates: a randomized controlled trial. Fertil Steril 2013. http://dx.doi.org/10.1016/j.fertnstert.2013.04.035.
44. Yang Z, Liu J, Collins GS, et al. Selection of single blastocysts for fresh transfer via standard morphology assessment alone and with array CGH for good prognosis IVF patients: results from a randomized pilot study. Mol Cytogenet 2012;5:24.
45. Harper JC, Wilton L, Traeger-Synodinos J, et al. The ESHRE PGD Consortium: 10 years of data collection. Hum Reprod Update 2012;18:234–47.

Uterine Factors

Carolyn R. Jaslow, PhD

KEYWORDS

- Recurrent miscarriage • Uterus • Septum • Fibroids • Uterine anomalies
- Pregnancy loss • Congenital • Acquired

KEY POINTS

- Uterine anomalies are one of the most common factors associated with recurrent pregnancy loss (RPL).
- Congenital anomalies, such as bicornuate, unicornuate, didelphic, and septate uteri, most likely result from HOX mutations in the developing Müllerian ducts.
- Of the acquired uterine anomalies, adhesions are typically formed after endometrial trauma, such as curettage, whereas fibroids and polyps are benign growths of the myometrium and endometrium, respectively.
- Many studies have explored the effects of uterine anomalies with respect to reproductive outcomes, but there are few randomized controlled trials, particularly for patients with RPL, and treatment methods lack strong supporting evidence.
- Nonetheless, metroplasty to correct a septate uterus and surgical removal of severe adhesions are recommended, and myomectomy of submucosal fibroids should be considered if no other causes have been identified.

INTRODUCTION

Recurrent pregnancy loss (RPL) is a frustrating disease that can cause considerable emotional distress in couples, often leading to a variety of other illnesses, both mental and physical.[1,2] Most often, RPL is caused by genetic abnormalities in the embryo[3]; nonetheless, chromosomal translocations, endocrine or metabolic disorders, autoimmune disorders, and anatomic anomalies of the uterus are considered the most likely parental causes associated with RPL.[4] Among the most prevalent of these parental factors are uterine anomalies, which are reported to occur in 19% of women with at least 2 consecutive miscarriages.[5] These anomalies include intrauterine adhesions, fibroids, and endometrial polyps that are acquired after birth, as well as congenital defects that arise from alterations in embryonic development, such as arcuate, bicornuate, didelphic, septate, T-shaped and unicornuate anomalies.

Disclosure: Nothing to disclose.
Department of Biology, Rhodes College, 2000 North Parkway, Memphis, TN 38112, USA
E-mail address: cjaslow@rhodes.edu

Obstet Gynecol Clin N Am 41 (2014) 57–86
http://dx.doi.org/10.1016/j.ogc.2013.10.002   obgyn.theclinics.com

IMAGING TO DIAGNOSE UTERINE ANOMALIES

Diagnostic testing for RPL causes can be costly and time consuming, but testing for anatomic abnormalities can bear the additional burden of subjecting a patient to an invasive procedure. Methods to identify uterine anomalies have included pelvic examination and dilation and curettage (D&C), hysterosalpingography (HSG), laparoscopy, laparotomy or other abdominal surgeries, two-dimensional or three-dimensional (3D) transabdominal or transvaginal ultrasonography alone or with saline infusion (sonohysterography [SHG]), magnetic resonance imagining (MRI), and hysteroscopy. Differences in sensitivity and specificity among these procedures have undoubtedly contributed to discrepancies in the literature regarding the prevalence and the reproductive consequences of uterine anomalies. Recent reviews identified 3D ultrasonography, SHG, hysteroscopy, and MRI as the most accurate procedures for diagnosis of uterine anomalies.[6–10] For detecting the separation of the uterine horns that distinguishes a bicornuate or didelphic uterus from a uterus with a partial or a complete septum, respectively, an external assessment of the uterus is needed. Thus, laparoscopy or laparotomy must accompany hysteroscopy for accurate diagnosis of these congenital anomalies.[6,7] Although hysteroscopy has the advantage of providing a direct view of the uterine cavity, and it can permit surgical correction of anomalies at the time of the procedure,[11] it is riskier and more invasive than the other imaging methods with high accuracy. Techniques such as MRI and 3D SHG are useful because they provide a recorded image of the anomaly, which can be saved and can allow subsequent measurements of the size and location of the anomaly.

NORMAL EMBRYOLOGY OF THE UTERUS

By the eighth week of gestation, the embryo has formed the paired Müllerian (paramesonephric) ducts that give rise to the oviducts, uterus, cervix, and the upper vagina.[12] Development of a single uterus starts with fusion of the Müllerian ducts near their caudal ends.[12] A septum initially separates the 2 ductal lumina, but it is gradually resorbed to produce a single uterine cavity.[12] This process may be controlled by uterine expression of Bcl-2, a protein that regulates apoptosis.[13] Case studies of women with a septate uterus and duplication of the cervix and vagina indicate that fusion begins at the developing uterine isthmus and progresses cranially and caudally simultaneously, followed by bidirectional resorption of the septum.[14] The unfused cranial portions of the 2 Müllerian ducts form the paired oviducts.

Based on studies of mice and other vertebrates, the Müllerian ducts originate from invagination of the coelomic epithelium lining the cranial end of the embryonic mesonephros.[15] These invaginating cells give rise to both the epithelium and the surrounding mesenchyme of the ducts, which canalize as they elongate caudally to contact the urogenital sinus.[14–16] The sites of invagination become the ostia of the oviducts, and the urogenital sinus becomes the lower vagina.[17] In the absence of testicular hormones (eg, anti–Müllerian hormone, testosterone), differentiation of the Müllerian ducts into the organs of the female reproductive tract involves reciprocal signaling between the duct epithelium and mesenchyme. Initially, the mesenchyme induces region-specific differentiation of the epithelium.[18] The epithelium then releases Wnt-7a signaling factors, which stimulate positional expression of a cluster of Hoxa genes located along the cranial-caudal axis of the mesenchyme, leading to proper morphogenesis of the oviducts, uterus, cervix, and upper vagina (**Box 1**).[19–21] In the uterus, the Müllerian duct epithelium forms the simple columnar epithelial lining and glands of the endometrium, and the mesenchyme forms the endometrial stroma and the myometrium.[18,22]

> **Box 1**
> **Cranial-caudal expression of the *HOXA* genes along the Müllerian ducts directs the development of the female reproductive organs**
>
> Oviduct - *HOXA9*
>
> Uterus - *HOXA10* and *HOXA11*
>
> Cervix - *HOXA11* and *HOXA13*
>
> Upper vagina - *HOXA13*.
>
> *Adapted from* Taylor HS, Vanden Heuvel GB, Igarashi P. A conserved Hox axis in the mouse and human female reproductive system: late establishment and persistent adult expression of the Hoxa cluster genes. Biol Reprod 1997;57:1341.

CONGENITAL UTERINE ANOMALIES
Classification and Embryology

Abnormalities in the formation, fusion, or differentiation of the Müllerian ducts, or in the regression of the septum, produce congenital uterine anomalies. The most common of these are the arcuate, bicornuate, didelphic, septate, T-shaped, and unicornuate forms (**Fig. 1**) defined by the American Fertility Society (AFS), now known as the American Society for Reproductive Medicine.[23] Agenetic defects may also occur, as can severe uterine hypoplasia, such as that associated with Mayer-Rokitansky-Kuster-Hauser syndrome,[24] but these anomalies are usually associated with amenorrhea or infertility, rather than RPL. Some studies have described other types of congenital anomalies and proposed alternative classification systems,[14,25] but the forms characterized by the AFS are the most prevalent, and their system is the most widely used.

Defects in formation of 1 Müllerian duct: unicornuate uterus
Agenesis or hypoplasia of 1 of the paired Müllerian ducts can result in a unicornuate uterus arising from the contralateral duct.[26] The term unicornuate implies that only 1 duct develops into a uterus; however, 74% of all unicornuate uteri have a rudimentary horn, which may or may not have a cavity, and may or may not communicate with the contralateral uterine cavity.[27] One complication of a rudimentary horn with a cavity is that it creates a site for an ectopic pregnancy, which can occur even in a noncommunicating rudimentary horn because of transperitoneal passage of sperm or fertilized ova.[28]

Defects in fusion of the Müllerian ducts: didelphic uterus and bicornuate uterus
A didelphic uterus forms if the 2 Müllerian ducts fail to fuse and each gives rise to a uterine horn with its own cervix (see **Fig. 1**).[29] A bicornuate uterus develops if the 2 Müllerian ducts fuse at their caudal regions, but remain separated at their cranial regions.[29] This situation creates 2 horns with connecting cavities and a common cervix (see **Fig. 1**). If the indentation between the 2 unfused horns of a bicornuate uterus extends to the cervix, the anomaly is a complete subtype.[23] A partial subtype can show a range of separation between the horns.[30]

Imaging techniques that show the V-shaped external contour of the fundus distinguish didelphic and bicornuate uteri from septate or arcuate anomalies. However, septate and arcuate uteri may have a minor degree of external indentation, so various quantitative criteria have been suggested to distinguish them from a partially bicornuate uterus. These criteria include the length or position of the indentation, or whether the angle it makes is acute or obtuse.[31–33]

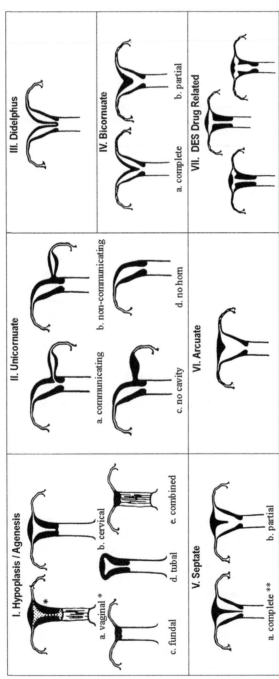

Fig. 1. Classification system of Müllerian duct anomalies. (*From* AFS. The American Fertility Society classifications of adnexal adhesions, distal tubal occlusion, tubal occlusion secondary to tubal ligation, tubal pregnancies, Müllerian anomalies and intrauterine adhesions. Fertil Steril 1988;49:952; with permission.)

Defects in regression of the septum: septate uterus and arcuate uterus
When the Müllerian ducts fuse completely and develop a normal external appearance, but the tissue between the 2 ducts is not resorbed, or is resorbed only partway, this creates a septate uterus (see **Fig. 1**).[29] A uterine septum is complete if it extends from the fundus through the cervix, or partial (subseptate) if it does not extend beyond the internal cervical os and permits communication between the 2 areas of the uterine cavity.[34,35] Histologic sections of septa show areas of irregularly organized smooth muscle, and also areas containing more connective tissue, particularly at the caudal tip of the septum.[32,36,37] Some aberrant vascular features have also been noted using MRI or histology.[30,37,38]

In an arcuate uterus, the internal fundus forms a broad but shallow bulge into the uterine cavity (see **Fig. 1**).[32] Many studies rely on this description for diagnosis, but others have proposed various criteria to quantify the projection.[39–42] There is no generally accepted formula. Some investigators describe a slight indentation of the external fundus and consider the arcuate uterus to be a mild form of a bicornuate uterus.[34,43] However, most studies characterize the fundal contour as normal, convex, or slightly flat,[23,30] which indicates that fusion of the 2 Müllerian ducts was complete and that the arcuate bulge is a small remnant of incomplete septal resorption. This explanation for the embryonic origin of an arcuate uterus is supported by MRI and sonographic data showing that the arcuate projection has muscular tissue like that in a partial septum.[30] It also has an unusual vascular pattern similar to the vascularization in a septum.[30] Inclusion of the arcuate form with other congenital uterine anomalies is controversial because some consider it a variation of normal uterine morphology, or at most, a minor anomaly.[23,30] Consequently, certain studies may include arcuate uteri in their reports of congenital anomalies, whereas others do not.[44–47]

Defects in differentiation of the Müllerian ducts: diethylstilbestrol drug-related uterus (T-shaped and hypoplastic)
Normally, the fused Müllerian ducts differentiate to form a uterus with a rounded cavity, but in patients exposed to diethylstilbestrol (DES) in utero, the uterine body becomes deformed, and the cavity becomes T-shaped and reduced in size (see **Fig. 1**).[48]

CAUSE
Environmental Factors

Because congenital uterine anomalies are uncommon and are often asymptomatic in the general population, identification of likely causes is challenging. A variety of environmental factors such as thalidomide, or exposure to infectious agents or ionizing radiation, have been suggested as possible teratogens,[43] but there is little evidence linking these environmental agents with the specific congenital uterine anomalies observed in women with RPL. In contrast, the effect of estrogenic endocrine disruptors on the development of T-shaped uterine anomalies is well documented, particularly for DES, a synthetic estrogen that was prescribed to prevent miscarriage in several million women from the 1940s until the 1970s.[19,48] Prenatal exposure to estrogenic endocrine disruptors such as DES affects uterine morphology by triggering changes in both the location and the amount of *HOXA/Hoxa* expression in the developing Müllerian duct.[49–51] Specifically, *Hoxa9* expression moves from the oviducts into the uterus, and *Hoxa10* and *Hoxa11* are expressed in different locations in the uterus, creating changes in the overall uterine form.[51]

- There are no known environmental causes for congenital uterine anomalies other than estrogenic endocrine disruptors such as DES.

Genetic Factors

Of 61 patients who had RPL and congenital uterine anomalies, only 1.9% had significant chromosomal rearrangements (eg, balanced translocations and mosaics).[45] This finding supports the assertion that most women with congenital uterine anomalies have a normal 46 XX karyotype,[43] and that any genetic basis for congenital uterine anomalies lies with mutations at the molecular level rather than with gross chromosomal rearrangements. For example, different types of *HOXA13* mutations cause congenital uterine defects that are part of hand-foot-genital syndrome.[52] More recently, a woman with a didelphic uterus was found to have a novel mutation in a *HOXA10* gene,[53] one of the *HOXA* genes responsible for normal uterine development (see **Box 1**). Furthermore, this mutation was shown to cause a functional amino acid substitution in the HOXA10 protein, which alters its ability to regulate other genes.[53] Despite this discovery, it is not yet clear how the altered HOXA10 protein might lead to a didelphic defect. Given the lack of direct connections between allelic sequence changes and most types of congenital uterine anomalies, and because only about 10% of uterine anomalies can be attributed to inheritance among families,[54] it seems that congenital uterine anomalies are most likely caused by a mix of different genes and epigenetic effects.[55]

- Congenital uterine anomalies are caused by HOX gene mutations, although the mechanism is most likely polygenic.
- Gross chromosomal rearrangements are unlikely to produce the congenital uterine anomalies associated with RPL.

PREVALENCE

Considerable variation exists among studies reporting the prevalence of congenital anomalies, in part because of a lack of consensus regarding the criteria used to define anomalies, and in part because some of the imaging methods used for diagnosis have low accuracy. **Table 1**A shows the results of a meta-analysis performed using only data that were collected with imaging techniques defined as highly accurate by Chan and colleagues[6] and Saravelos and colleagues.[7] Congenital uterine anomalies (arcuate, bicornuate, didelphic, septate, T-shaped, and unicornuate types) were found in 16.4% of women with RPL. When arcuate uteri were excluded because they may be considered a normal form or a minor variant, this value decreased to about 8.4% (see **Table 1**B). Even without arcuate forms, the 8.4% rate of uterine anomalies was 7 times greater than the frequency of 1.2% among women in the general population, a rate that is likely an overestimation because it includes women presenting with pelvic pain and abnormal bleeding.[7] A recent review reported that women who had a history of miscarriage had significantly greater rates of congenital anomalies compared with women in unselected populations.[6]

Table 2 lists the prevalence of specific types of congenital anomalies among women with RPL compared with rates reported for the general population by systematic reviews.[6,7] The data for women with RPL are derived from meta-analyses of studies that used 3D ultrasonography, SHG, or hysteroscopy and laparoscopy for diagnosis (**Table 3**). The T-shaped uterus is not included here because its prevalence is linked to exposure to DES, which was discontinued after 1971. A septate uterus is the most common type of congenital anomaly among patients with RPL (6.1%). For bicornuate, septate, and unicornuate anomalies, the prevalence among patients with RPL is at least twice that in the general population. The frequency of didelphic uteri does not differ between groups, perhaps because the rates reported in the

Table 1

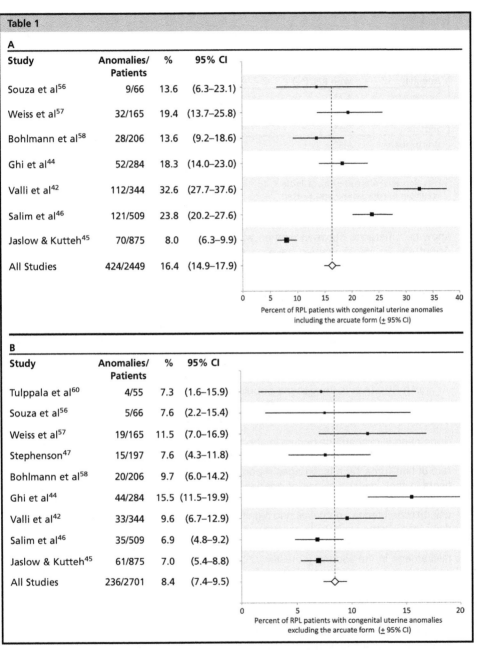

A

Study	Anomalies/ Patients	%	95% CI
Souza et al[56]	9/66	13.6	(6.3–23.1)
Weiss et al[57]	32/165	19.4	(13.7–25.8)
Bohlmann et al[58]	28/206	13.6	(9.2–18.6)
Ghi et al[44]	52/284	18.3	(14.0–23.0)
Valli et al[42]	112/344	32.6	(27.7–37.6)
Salim et al[46]	121/509	23.8	(20.2–27.6)
Jaslow & Kutteh[45]	70/875	8.0	(6.3–9.9)
All Studies	424/2449	16.4	(14.9–17.9)

Percent of RPL patients with congenital uterine anomalies including the arcuate form (± 95% CI)

B

Study	Anomalies/ Patients	%	95% CI
Tulppala et al[60]	4/55	7.3	(1.6–15.9)
Souza et al[56]	5/66	7.6	(2.2–15.4)
Weiss et al[57]	19/165	11.5	(7.0–16.9)
Stephenson[47]	15/197	7.6	(4.3–11.8)
Bohlmann et al[58]	20/206	9.7	(6.0–14.2)
Ghi et al[44]	44/284	15.5	(11.5–19.9)
Valli et al[42]	33/344	9.6	(6.7–12.9)
Salim et al[46]	35/509	6.9	(4.8–9.2)
Jaslow & Kutteh[45]	61/875	7.0	(5.4–8.8)
All Studies	236/2701	8.4	(7.4–9.5)

Percent of RPL patients with congenital uterine anomalies excluding the arcuate form (± 95% CI)

Prevalence of all congenital uterine anomalies with (*A*), and without (*B*) arcuate anomalies among patients with RPL. Studies were included if they had subjects with 2 or more or 3 or more miscarriages, reported the frequency for all types of congenital anomalies, and used 3D ultrasonography, SHG, or hysteroscopy and laparoscopy for diagnosis. Forest plots were generated with the MIX 2.0 Pro software for meta-analysis in Excel, which used the Freeman-Tukey double arcsine transformation to calculate the 95% confidence intervals, weights, and the prevalence proportions for each study and for the summary of all studies.[59]

Table 2
Prevalence of congenital uterine anomalies in women with RPL and women in the general population

Anomaly	Prevalence in Patients with RPL (%)	Prevalence in the General Population (%)[6,7]
Bicornuate	1.2[a]	0.3–0.4
Didelphic	0.2[b]	0.03–0.3
Septate	6.1[a]	2.0–2.3
Unicornuate	0.5[a]	0.03–0.1
Arcuate	4.6[a]	3.9–4.9

[a] Prevalence of all studies from **Table 3**.
[b] Prevalence from Jaslow and Kutteh.[45]

2 reviews of the general population vary by an order of magnitude. Arcuate uteri also show no difference between women with RPL and those in the general population. About 4% to 5% of women have an arcuate uterus, irrespective of whether they have RPL; however, there is a considerable variation among studies reporting the prevalence of an arcuate uterus in patients with RPL (see **Table 3**D). Most likely, this variation reflects the difficulty of distinguishing an arcuate uterus from a normal uterus if the arcuate projection is small, or from a subseptate (or possibly bicornuate) uterus if the arcuate projection is large. It is also possible that the prevalence of arcuate and didelphic uteri do not differ between women with early RPL and the general population because neither uterine anomaly represents a cause for early RPL.

- Congenital anomalies, particularly septate uteri, are more prevalent in women with RPL than in the general population.

CONGENITAL ANOMALIES AND FIRST-TRIMESTER PREGNANCY LOSS

Spontaneous miscarriage occurs in about 11% to 15% of clinical pregnancies among women in the general population.[62,63] This finding is comparable with the 13% to 15% rate of first-trimester miscarriages reported by Chan and colleagues[64] for control patients in their meta-analyses of congenital uterine anomalies and reproductive outcomes. In this study, patients with septate (including subseptate), bicornuate, and unicornuate uterine anomalies had significantly greater risks of first-trimester miscarriage than did the controls. In contrast, arcuate and didelphic uteri did not increase the first-trimester miscarriage risk, although arcuate anomalies did increase the risk of miscarriage in the second trimester. Other studies have reported similar patterns in which higher rates of first-trimester miscarriage occurred in women with septate, unicornuate, or bicornuate anomalies compared with those with arcuate, didelphic, or normal uteri (**Table 4**).[40,65–67] These results support the argument that arcuate and didelphic uterine forms do not contribute to the likelihood of early RPL, but that septate, unicornuate, and bicornuate anomalies may warrant further consideration in patients presenting with at least 2 consecutive early losses.

One limitation of these studies is that they did not restrict their sample population to patients with RPL. In the 1 study that included only women with 3 or more consecutive losses,[68] the frequency of first-trimester miscarriages in a subsequent pregnancy was higher than among women in the general population, but the rates did not differ based on the type of congenital anomaly (see **Table 4**). Because women with congenital anomalies do not always experience diminished reproductive outcomes, it is reasonable that the miscarriage rate would be lower for the general population than for

Table 3

A

Study	Anomalies/Patients	%	95% CI	
Weiss et al[57]	3/165	1.8	(0.2–4.6)	
Stephenson[47]	1/197	0.5	(0.4–2.2)	
Bohlmann et al[58]	5/206	2.4	(0.7–5.1)	
Ghi et al[44]	8/284	2.8	(1.2–5.1)	
Salim et al[46]	6/509	1.2	(0.4–2.3)	
Jaslow & Kutteh[45]	7/875	0.8	(0.3–1.5)	
All Studies	30/2236	1.2	(0.8–1.7)	

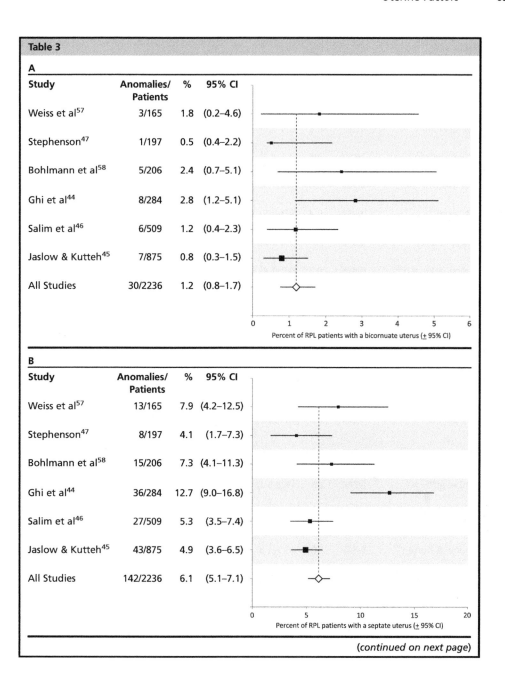

Percent of RPL patients with a bicornuate uterus (± 95% CI)

B

Study	Anomalies/Patients	%	95% CI	
Weiss et al[57]	13/165	7.9	(4.2–12.5)	
Stephenson[47]	8/197	4.1	(1.7–7.3)	
Bohlmann et al[58]	15/206	7.3	(4.1–11.3)	
Ghi et al[44]	36/284	12.7	(9.0–16.8)	
Salim et al[46]	27/509	5.3	(3.5–7.4)	
Jaslow & Kutteh[45]	43/875	4.9	(3.6–6.5)	
All Studies	142/2236	6.1	(5.1–7.1)	

Percent of RPL patients with a septate uterus (± 95% CI)

(continued on next page)

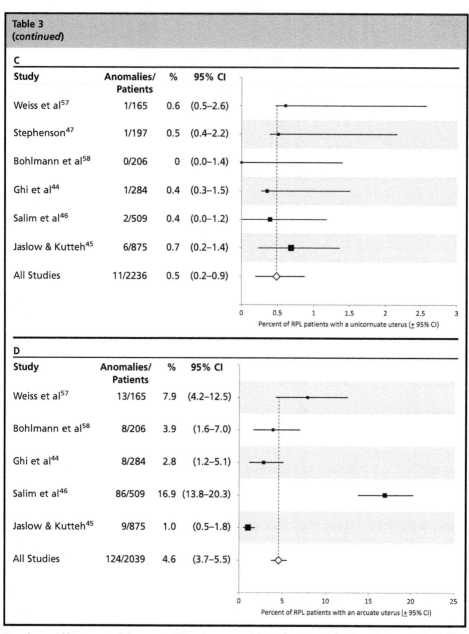

Table 3
(continued)

C

Study	Anomalies/ Patients	%	95% CI
Weiss et al[57]	1/165	0.6	(0.5–2.6)
Stephenson[47]	1/197	0.5	(0.4–2.2)
Bohlmann et al[58]	0/206	0	(0.0–1.4)
Ghi et al[44]	1/284	0.4	(0.3–1.5)
Salim et al[46]	2/509	0.4	(0.0–1.2)
Jaslow & Kutteh[45]	6/875	0.7	(0.2–1.4)
All Studies	11/2236	0.5	(0.2–0.9)

Percent of RPL patients with a unicornuate uterus (± 95% CI)

D

Study	Anomalies/ Patients	%	95% CI
Weiss et al[57]	13/165	7.9	(4.2–12.5)
Bohlmann et al[58]	8/206	3.9	(1.6–7.0)
Ghi et al[44]	8/284	2.8	(1.2–5.1)
Salim et al[46]	86/509	16.9	(13.8–20.3)
Jaslow & Kutteh[45]	9/875	1.0	(0.5–1.8)
All Studies	124/2039	4.6	(3.7–5.5)

Percent of RPL patients with an arcuate uterus (± 95% CI)

Prevalence of bicornuate (A), septate (B), unicornuate (C), and arcuate (D) types of congenital uterine anomalies, among studies of patients with RPL. Studies were included if they had subjects with 2 or more or 3 or more miscarriages and used 3D ultrasonography, SHG, or hysteroscopy and laparoscopy for diagnosis. Forest plots were generated with the MIX 2.0 Pro software for meta-analysis in Excel, which used the Freeman-Tukey double arcsine transformation to calculate the 95% confidence intervals, weights, and the prevalence proportions for each study with prevalence greater than 0% and for the summary of all studies.[59] The upper 95% CI was calculated as $1-0.05^{1/n}$ for investigations with prevalence of 0%.[61]

Table 4
Frequency of pregnancies ending in first-trimester miscarriage among women with
congenital uterine anomalies in 2 different study populations

Anomaly	Rates for All Women (%)	Rates for Only Women with RPL (%)[68]
Bicornuate	38[64]	72
Didelphic	11[64]	80
Septate	34[64]	73
Unicornuate	20–24[26,64]	60
Arcuate	15–20[a]	73

Abbreviation: RPL, Recurrent pregnancy loss, defined by Saravelos and colleagues[68] as ≥3 consecutive miscarriages.
[a] The rate of 15% excludes 1 study that had a miscarriage rate (34%) more than double that reported by the other 4 studies in the review (14%–16%).[64]

women with RPL. Further research is needed to confirm the pattern of the first-trimester miscarriage rates among the different types of congenital defects in women with RPL, particularly because the rates for the didelphic and unicornuate anomalies were based on pregnancies for only 1 patient in each category.

- The likelihood of first-trimester miscarriage is higher in women with septate, bicornuate, or unicornuate uterine anomalies than among women in the general population, particularly if the women also have a history of RPL.

POSSIBLE MECHANISMS CAUSING MISCARRIAGE

First-trimester miscarriage is a risk for women with congenital uterine anomalies, but little is known about the mechanisms responsible, which may be different from those acting to cause miscarriage later during pregnancy. For example, 2 factors suggested to cause reduced pregnancy outcomes in women with congenital uterine anomalies are cervical incompetence and reduced muscle in the myometrium.[26] However, these are doubtful causes for early RPL because they would be more likely to cause problems when fetal size is greater during the latter part of a pregnancy. In 1 study of women with a septate uterus, first-trimester miscarriage occurred more often among embryos implanted on the septum than those implanted elsewhere on the uterine walls.[69] Histologic studies comparing the septum with the other uterine walls found differences in the proportion of connective tissue relative to muscle, and in vascularization and endometrial structure, all of which could play a role in miscarriage.[37,38,70]

Altered uterine blood flow is another factor believed to cause pregnancy loss in women with congenital uterine anomalies,[34] and different types of studies provide support for this hypothesis. Doppler ultrasonography showed different uterine blood flow and perfusion in pregnant women who subsequently experienced first-trimester miscarriages, and in those who had congenital uterine anomalies.[71,72] Dye tracings in the uterine vasculature showed that women with bifurcated uterine arteries had experienced more miscarriages compared with women who had normal single arteries, although it was not stated whether these losses were early or late.[73] Possibly, the absence or modification of the uterine arteries in a unicornuate uterus or a uterus with a fusion defect causes a change in blood flow, which leads to first-trimester pregnancy loss.[74]

- More research is needed to identify how congenital uterine anomalies cause first-trimester miscarriage, but alterations in vascularization and blood flow may be factors.

TREATMENT OPTIONS
Metroplasty

Unicornuate uterus
Metroplasty is not recommended for a unicornuate uterus, although surgical removal of an existing rudimentary horn is recommended to reduce dysmenorrhea and other menstrual complications, and to avoid the risk of an ectopic pregnancy.[29]

Bicornuate uterus
Previously, surgical repair of a bicornuate uterus was recommended for women with RPL, but only if other factors for miscarriage were ruled out.[75–77] A transabdominal metroplasty was traditionally used to effect uterine repair,[76] but studies have reported success performing this surgery laparoscopically.[75] Because of the invasiveness of this procedure and the paucity of clinical studies showing improved outcomes, surgical repair of a bicornuate uterus is seldom performed in the United States.

Didelphic uterus
Some investigators recommend treating a didelphic uterus the same way as a bicornuate uterus by performing metroplasty only in women with RPL for whom no other cause can be identified.[75,76] Others believe that surgical correction is unlikely to improve reproductive outcome.[29,78] It remains unclear whether surgical correction is warranted in women with RPL who have a didelphic uterus.

Septate uterus
Although there are no randomized controlled trials,[79] reviews have shown that hysteroscopic removal of a complete or partial uterine septum produces substantial reductions in miscarriage rates among women with RPL, as well as among women with RPL and other obstetric complications.[31,80,81] In most cases, these investigations report pregnancy rates or rates of spontaneous abortions without clarification whether the losses occurred in the first trimester or later. This situation makes it more difficult to assess the benefit of septum resection specifically for patients with RPL in the first trimester, although a single study[82] did find that first-trimester miscarriage rates in these patients dropped from 96% to 16% after hysteroscopic metroplasty of the septum.

Arcuate uterus
The effect of an arcuate uterus on reproductive success is controversial, as is the question of whether to recommend surgical removal. One review stated directly that "women with such anomalies do not benefit from surgical intervention,"[34] and others have not recommended surgery because they do not believe that arcuate anomalies affect reproductive outcome.[77,83] Although some studies found that miscarriage rate declined after arcuate metroplasty, none separated first-trimester losses from later ones.[39,84–86] Because women with an arcuate uterus have a higher frequency of second-trimester miscarriages compared with women who have a normal uterus,[40,64] arcuate metroplasty appears to have little advantage for a patient who is suffering from first-trimester RPL.

Cervical Cerclage

Cerclage of the cervix has been reported to improve reproductive outcomes for patients with a range of congenital uterine anomalies,[87] although randomized, controlled studies are lacking.[26] In most cases, cervical cerclage is noted as a solution for late-trimester losses and preterm births rather than for resolving first-trimester miscarriages.

- For women with early RPL who have congenital uterine anomalies, there is an absence of randomized controlled trials comparing the effect of surgical correction with expectant management; nonetheless, metroplasty is recommended for women who have a septate uterus, and it may be considered as a last resort for women with a bicornuate uterus if no other causes have been identified.

ACQUIRED UTERINE ANOMALIES

Acquired uterine anomalies associated with RPL include intrauterine adhesions, fibroids, and endometrial polyps. These anomalies develop after puberty, often because of some physical or hormonal stimulus. Acquired anomalies occur in about 12% of women with RPL, but this frequency ranges widely from 1% to 33% (**Table 5**A). This variation is most likely the result of differences and ambiguity in criteria for diagnosis, particularly for adhesions.

Adhesions

Characteristics and classification

Intrauterine adhesions connect opposing walls of the uterus. At one extreme, they are sites where the uterine walls have fused, obliterating all or parts of the uterine cavity and the normal functional and basal layers of the endometrium.[94,95] For women with RPL, adhesions more likely are bands of tissue extending from wall to wall (called fibrosis by Yu and colleagues[95]). These adhesions may be thin strands of endometrial tissue, fibromuscular connections covered with abnormal endometrium (these are the most commonly observed), or bands of fibrous connective tissue with no endometrial covering.[95–97] In 1988, the AFS published a system that classified the type of adhesion (filmy to dense), the extent of the cavity involved (from <one-third to >two-thirds), and an assessment of the patient's menstrual pattern (normal to amenorrheic).[23] Others have proposed different classifications, some of which include information about the histology of the adhesions or the reproductive performance of the patient, but none has been used consistently.[97,98]

Cause

Adhesions arise after destruction of the regenerating basal layer of the endometrium.[99,100] In a study of 1856 cases of adhesions, more than 90% occurred in patients who had experienced curettage during induced abortions or for complications after birth or spontaneous abortions.[99] Further evidence comes from prospective studies that reported adhesions in 19% to 40% of patients examined hysteroscopically after curettage.[101,102] In addition to curettage, infection with genital tuberculosis can cause adhesions, and uterine surgery or other traumas (eg, myomectomy) are possible causes.[99]

Some predisposing factors for adhesions include infections and heredity, but the foremost factor is pregnancy, probably because it makes the endometrium vulnerable to physical trauma so that curettage more easily removes or damages the basal layer.[96,99] Another hypothesis is that the decrease in estrogen level with loss of the placenta at birth or miscarriage plays a role, because estrogen stimulates regeneration of the endometrial basal layer.[95] Schenker and Margalioth[99] noted that adhesions were more likely to arise when curettage was performed between 2 and 4 weeks post partum, possibly related to hormonal changes.[100] Another key factor believed to predispose women to develop adhesions is the retention of products of conception in the uterus after pregnancy or during a missed abortion.[99,100]

Table 5

A

Study	Anomalies/ Patients	%	95% CI	
Ventolini et al[88]	7/23	30.4	(13.0–51.0)	
Dendrinos et al[89]	15/48	31.3	(18.8–45.2)	
Tulppala et al[60]	7/55	12.7	(5.0–23.0)	
Guimarães Filho et al[90]	19/58	32.8	(21.2–45.4)	
Souza et al[56]	13/66	19.7	(10.9–30.3)	
Cogendez et al[91]	18/82	22.0	(13.6–31.6)	
Raziel et al[92]	27/106	25.5	(17.6–34.2)	
Weiss et al[57]	18/165	10.9	(6.6–16.2)	
Stephenson[47]	12/197	6.1	(3.1–9.9)	
Bohlmann et al[58]	58/206	28.2	(22.2–34.5)	
Coulam[93]	2/214	0.9	(0.0–2.8)	
Valli et al[42]	30/344	8.7	(6.0–12.0)	
Jaslow & Kutteh[45]	113/875	12.9	(10.8–15.2)	
All Studies	339/2439	12.5	(11.2–13.8)	

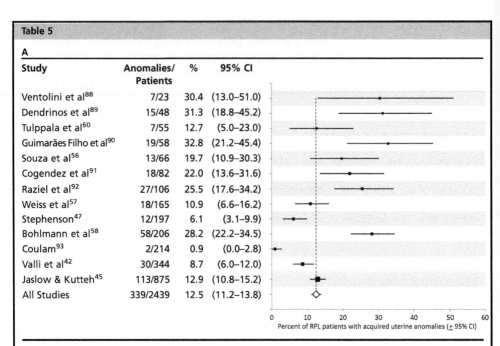

Percent of RPL patients with acquired uterine anomalies (± 95% CI)

B

Study	Anomalies/ Patients	%	95% CI	
Ventolini et al[88]	5/23	21.7	(6.9–41.2)	
Dendrinos et al[89]	9/48	18.8	(8.8–31.2)	
Tulppala et al[60]	5/55	9.1	(2.7–18.4)	
Guimarães Filho et al[90]	16/58	27.6	(16.8–39.9)	
Souza et al[56]	7/66	10.6	(4.1–19.3)	
Cogendez et al[91]	10/82	12.2	(5.9–20.3)	
Raziel et al[92]	25/106	23.6	(15.9–32.2)	
Weiss et al[57]	11/165	6.7	(3.3–11.0)	
Stephenson[47]	11/197	5.6	(2.8–9.3)	
Bohlmann et al[58]	26/206	12.6	(8.4–17.5)	
Coulam[93]	1/214	0.5	(0.4–2.0)	
Valli et al[42]	15/344	4.4	(2.4–6.8)	
Li et al[104]	17/453	3.8	(2.2–5.7)	
Jaslow & Kutteh[45]	36/875	4.1	(2.9–5.5)	
All Studies	194/2892	5.5	(4.7–6.4)	

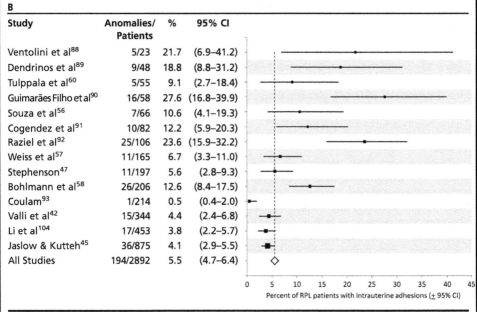

Percent of RPL patients with intrauterine adhesions (± 95% CI)

(continued on next page)

Table 5
(continued)

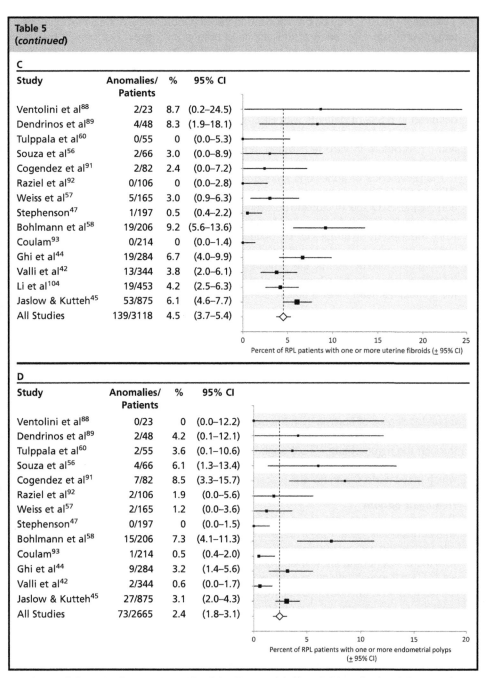

C

Study	Anomalies/ Patients	%	95% CI
Ventolini et al[88]	2/23	8.7	(0.2–24.5)
Dendrinos et al[89]	4/48	8.3	(1.9–18.1)
Tulppala et al[60]	0/55	0	(0.0–5.3)
Souza et al[56]	2/66	3.0	(0.0–8.9)
Cogendez et al[91]	2/82	2.4	(0.0–7.2)
Raziel et al[92]	0/106	0	(0.0–2.8)
Weiss et al[57]	5/165	3.0	(0.9–6.3)
Stephenson[47]	1/197	0.5	(0.4–2.2)
Bohlmann et al[58]	19/206	9.2	(5.6–13.6)
Coulam[93]	0/214	0	(0.0–1.4)
Ghi et al[44]	19/284	6.7	(4.0–9.9)
Valli et al[42]	13/344	3.8	(2.0–6.1)
Li et al[104]	19/453	4.2	(2.5–6.3)
Jaslow & Kutteh[45]	53/875	6.1	(4.6–7.7)
All Studies	139/3118	4.5	(3.7–5.4)

Percent of RPL patients with one or more uterine fibroids (± 95% CI)

D

Study	Anomalies/ Patients	%	95% CI
Ventolini et al[88]	0/23	0	(0.0–12.2)
Dendrinos et al[89]	2/48	4.2	(0.1–12.1)
Tulppala et al[60]	2/55	3.6	(0.1–10.6)
Souza et al[56]	4/66	6.1	(1.3–13.4)
Cogendez et al[91]	7/82	8.5	(3.3–15.7)
Raziel et al[92]	2/106	1.9	(0.0–5.6)
Weiss et al[57]	2/165	1.2	(0.0–3.6)
Stephenson[47]	0/197	0	(0.0–1.5)
Bohlmann et al[58]	15/206	7.3	(4.1–11.3)
Coulam[93]	1/214	0.5	(0.4–2.0)
Ghi et al[44]	9/284	3.2	(1.4–5.6)
Valli et al[42]	2/344	0.6	(0.0–1.7)
Jaslow & Kutteh[45]	27/875	3.1	(2.0–4.3)
All Studies	73/2665	2.4	(1.8–3.1)

Percent of RPL patients with one or more endometrial polyps (± 95% CI)

Prevalence of all acquired uterine anomalies (*A*), adhesions (*B*), fibroids (*C*), and polyps (*D*) among studies of patients with RPL. Studies were included if they had subjects with 2 or more or 3 or more miscarriages, reported the frequency of all types of acquired anomalies, and used 3D ultrasonography SHG, or hysteroscopy for diagnosis. Forest plots were generated with the MIX 2.0 Pro software for meta-analysis in Excel, which used the Freeman-Tukey double arcsine transformation to calculate the 95% confidence intervals, weights, and the prevalence proportions for each study with prevalence >0% and for the summary of all studies.[59] The upper 95% CI was calculated as $1-0.05^{1/n}$ for investigations with prevalence of 0%.[61]

Women with RPL may be predisposed to develop intrauterine adhesions if they undergo curettage after each of their multiple pregnancy losses. Not only is the frequency of adhesions higher in women with 2 or more postabortion curettages compared with those with only 1 procedure, but the adhesions are more severe.[101,103]

Prevalence

A meta-analysis of studies that used SHG or hysteroscopy showed that adhesions occurred in 5.5% of patients with RPL (see **Table 5**B). In contrast, adhesions were detected in 1.5% to 3% of women who had a hysteroscopy before tubal sterilization,[105] or before in vitro fertilization (IVF) for idiopathic or male factor infertility, or for problems unrelated to uterine anomalies (eg, tubal factors).[106,107]

The prevalence of adhesions among the studies in **Table 5**B ranged widely, from 0.5% to 28%. Some of this variation may be attributed to differences in classification and diagnosis. Of the 14 studies represented, only 5 describe the criteria used to report adhesions. In 1982, Schenker and Margalioth[99] suggested that the prevalence of adhesions reported by 90 studies varied because of different diagnostic criteria used by clinicians in various locations, as well as their awareness of the problem. These investigators also noted that there might be regional differences in some of the causes for adhesions, such as the frequency of elective abortions (particularly illegal abortions), the techniques used for evacuation, and the prevalence of genital tuberculosis.[99]

First-trimester pregnancy loss

A 1982 review reported a miscarriage rate of 40% for 7 studies of women with adhesions, although the investigations were not restricted to patients with RPL.[99] Miscarriage may occur because adhesions diminish the available uterine space and restrict expansion[99]; however, these limitations may not be as important in the first trimester as later in pregnancy. In a uterus with adhesions, the endometrium may be abnormal or it may be replaced by fibrous connective tissue, and the myometrium may also have a greater degree of fibrosis than the myometrium of a normal uterus.[108,109] Uteri with adhesions may also have diminished vascular density, which reduces blood flow through the myometrium,[110] although it is not clear if this occurs as a consequence of fibrosis. Collectively, these factors reduce the amount of functional endometrium, which may interfere with normal placental invasion and development.[95,99,109]

Treatment options

There are no studies that assess the success of expectant management compared with adhesiolysis, other than a review from 1982,[99] which reported a 40% miscarriage rate for women without surgery and a 25% rate for women who had surgery. Reviews with more recent data show miscarriage rates of about 15% to 16% after adhesiolysis.[95,100] In 2 investigations, miscarriage rates after surgery were reported separately for patients with infertility and for those with pregnancy loss (defined as pregnancy wastage or $\geq$3 losses).[97,111] Women with pregnancy loss had a miscarriage rate of only 10% (10/103) after surgery, compared with a rate of 30% (24/79) for infertile women, which suggests that adhesiolysis might be a more effective treatment for women with RPL than for women with other reproductive problems.

The treatment of adhesions is surgical removal, but because uterine surgery is a cause for adhesions in the first place, the techniques used should seek to prevent recurrence of the adhesions and to facilitate endometrial regeneration.[95] Recent thorough reviews summarize some of the advantages and disadvantages of these methods, which include different instruments used to lyse adhesions, methods of guidance, physical barriers to prevent contact between the walls after lysis, and hormone treatments to stimulate endometrial regeneration.[94,95,100]

- Damage to the endometrium via curettage is the predominant cause of adhesions. This damage may increase the risk of adhesions for women with RPL if their multiple pregnancy losses cause them to undergo repeated curettage.
- The reported prevalence of adhesions is highly variable, possibly because of differences in diagnosis or the causes among study groups.
- Women with adhesions seem to have a high rate of miscarriages, but the supporting evidence for this is limited.
- Although there is a great need for randomized controlled studies of this issue, surgical removal of adhesions should be recommended for women with RPL who have no other known causes, with great precaution taken to prevent recurrence.

Fibroids (Leiomyomata)

Characteristics and classification

Fibroids are benign smooth muscle tumors that originate in the myometrium and may grow to invade other parts of the uterus. Several reviews (eg, Ciarmela and colleagues[112] and Flake and colleagues[113]) have described a range of fibroid cellular and extracellular properties, some of which are summarized in **Box 2**.

Fibroids are typically classified according to their anatomic position[123]:

- Submucosal fibroids distort the uterine cavity and may be subdivided based on whether they are pedunculated, have less than 50% intramural penetration, or 50% or more intramural penetration.

Box 2
Cellular and extracellular characteristics of fibroids compared with myometrial tissue, and some examples of the functions or significance of these features

1. Fibroids contain abnormal myocytes and a large amount of aberrant extracellular matrix (ECM)[114,115]

    - eg, the abnormal fibroid ECM, composed of fibroblasts, collagen, fibronectin, and proteoglycans, is a source of signaling factors and mediators that communicate with the smooth muscle cells of the fibroid to promote growth.[116,117]

2. Fibroids have different densities of receptors for estrogen, progesterone, and growth factors[113,118]

    - eg, an altered ratio of alpha and beta estrogen receptors in fibroids compared with myometrium may promote estrogen-stimulated fibroid growth.[119]

3. Fibroid cellular and extracellular proteins and enzymes are expressed in different quantities and have different levels of activity

    - eg, reduced activity of 17β-hydroxysteroid dehydrogenase, which converts estradiol to the less potent estrone,[118] likely contributes to fibroid growth. Recently, proteomic techniques have identified several other fibroid proteins and enzymes that have altered expression compared with myometrium.[120]

4. Fibroids express different quantities of growth factors

    - eg, platelet-derived growth factor C (PDGFC) is one of the many growth factors that are overexpressed and thus promote growth in fibroids.[121]

5. Fibroids may show degenerative changes

    - eg, degenerative features such as hyaline deposits, calcification, and hemorrhage may appear in large fibroids, presumably because they have outgrown their blood supply.[122]

- Intramural fibroids do not distort the uterine cavity and do not extend more than halfway through the serosal surface of the uterus.
- Subserosal fibroids extend 50% or more through the serosal surface and may be pedunculated.

Cause and development

Risk factors linked with fibroids include nulliparity, early onset of menarche, increased age, obesity, and African American ethnicity.[113] In addition, about 50% of surgically removed fibroids have gross chromosomal rearrangements, particularly a translocation between chromosomes 12 and 14 (t(12;14)(q14-15;q23–24)), a deletion on chromosome 7 (del(7)(q22q32)), and various alterations on chromosome 6 (6p21)[113,124] Some of these cytogenetic anomalies vary with fibroid location[125] and size,[126] and molecular analyses have found regulatory genes with the potential to affect fibroid growth (eg, *HMG*) located in or near the regions of the chromosomal abnormalities.[113,124] Furthermore, fibroids can show epigenetic markers that likely contributed to their development, such as altered DNA methylation in the promoter region of an estrogen receptor that increased expression of the receptor.[117,127]

The development of fibroids includes the formation of an abnormal myometrial cell, followed by proliferation of that cell into a benign tumor.[128] It is established that proliferation of cells to form a fibroid is driven by exposure to estrogen and progesterone and is regulated by several autocrine growth factors, other signaling molecules (eg, interleukins), and components of the extracellular matrix (see **Box 2** and comprehensive reviews[113,117]). On the other hand, the factors responsible for the transformation of a normal cell to an abnormal one, possibly with some of the genetic or epigenetic anomalies listed earlier, are less clearly understood.

Some hypotheses for the initiation of a fibroid, summarized by Flake and colleagues,[113] propose that individuals with higher levels of estrogen and progesterone, or more receptors for those hormones, have a greater risk for somatic mutations in their myometrium because estrogen and progesterone increase the rate of mitosis. It has also been suggested that the appearance of a cell with a tendency to proliferate may be a response to hypoxia during menstrual vasoconstriction.[113]

Evidence supporting a heritable basis for fibroid development derives from epidemiologic studies of fibroids in families and in groups with different racial ethnicity.[124] Close family members of women with fibroids have more than double the risk of developing fibroids themselves,[129] and African American women are about 3 times more likely to develop fibroids than White women, irrespective of other factors such as age, body mass index, parity, and so forth.[130,131] More recently, searches for the mutations underlying these patterns of inheritance have identified specific heritable genetic polymorphisms associated with development of fibroids in some populations of women.[132,133]

Prevalence

A meta-analysis of studies that used SHG or hysteroscopy found fibroids in 4.5% of the patients with RPL (see **Table 5C**). This analysis included only submucosal fibroids, defined earlier as fibroids that distort the uterine cavity. Commonly cited studies of fibroid prevalence have reported frequencies of 70% or more among the general population, but those rates include all fibroids, regardless of size or location.[130,134] When 1 study[130] tallied only the clinically relevant fibroids (eg, submucosal fibroids, or fibroids ≥4 cm in diameter), the prevalence declined to 35% to 50%. Another consideration of these studies is that they measured fibroids in patients who were predominantly

30 to 50 years of age.[130,134] The prevalence of fibroids increases with age among pre-menopausal women,[130,131] so greater frequencies of fibroids are likely to occur among women in these older cohorts than among women seeking treatment of RPL, whose mean age is about 29 to 34 years.[5,57,58,91] Fibroid prevalence among younger women in the general population is only 5% to 15%,[135–137] and 1 study that reported the breakdown of different fibroid types among 101 women 18 to 30 years old observed no submucosal fibroids.[137] Compared with this finding, a rate of 4.5% submucosal fibroids among women with RPL is increased.

First-trimester pregnancy loss

Two systematic reviews reported that submucosal fibroids significantly increase the rate of miscarriages.[138,139] Although neither review specified whether the losses occurred in the first trimester or later, the miscarriage rate for women with fibroids was as high as 47%.[138] Both reviews also reported that miscarriage rates were increased in women with intramural fibroids; however, when studies using less accurate diagnostic techniques were excluded in 1 review, no effect was seen.[139] No effect of intramural fibroids on miscarriage rate was found in a systematic review of women undergoing IVF.[140] Among women with RPL who had fibroids distorting the uterine cavity, 42% of pregnancies ended in first-trimester loss.[141]

The mechanisms by which fibroids might trigger first-trimester miscarriage are not known. One hypothesis is that the abnormal ultrastructural properties of myocytes in fibroids and the surrounding myometrium might cause irregular contractions, which lead to pregnancy loss.[114] Most studies have focused instead on endometrial changes that contribute to implantation failure and infertility (**Box 3**), but it is possible that some of these changes may play a role in disrupting pregnancy in women with RPL. An underlying fibroid may exert a deleterious effect on the endometrium either through a mechanical stimulus, if the fibroid impinges on the cavity, or a molecular one, such as the inhibitory effect of fibroid transforming growth factor β_3 on endometrial expression of molecules involved in implantation.[142,143]

Treatment options

The options for treatment of fibroids depend on the location, number, and size of the fibroids, and on the desire of the patient for future reproductive opportunities.[8] Because subserosal and intramural fibroids are not considered likely factors contributing to RPL, this section focuses only on treatment of submucosal fibroids, defined earlier as fibroids that project into the uterine cavity, with or without intramural penetration. Hysterectomy and medical therapies are not included, because neither is considered an option for a woman who desires future fertility.[8]

Box 3

Examples of endometrial changes that contribute to implantation failure and infertility in uteri with fibroids as reviewed by Makker and Goel[144]

- Altered expression of cytokines and other regulatory molecules and receptors (eg, thrombomodulin)[143]

- Accumulation of inflammatory cells (eg, macrophages)[145]

- Architectural changes (eg, degeneration of glandular structure)[142]

Data from Makker A, Goel MM. Uterine leiomyomas: effects on architectural, cellular, and molecular determinants of endometrial receptivity. Reprod Sci 2013;20:631–8.

Myomectomy is the surgery commonly recommended for women with symptomatic submucosal fibroids who also wish to bear a child[146]; however, there is conflicting evidence whether myomectomy can significantly reduce the risk of pregnancy loss in women with RPL. Of 3 studies that compared the rate of first-trimester miscarriage (<12 weeks) in women with RPL before and after myomectomy, 2 reported significant declines in miscarriage rate, but the third found no difference.[141,147,148] According to a recent Cochrane review, there is only 1 randomized controlled trial that has examined the effect of myomectomy on first-trimester miscarriage rate.[149] In this study of 94 infertile women with submucosal fibroids 4 cm or less, women who had undergone a myomectomy experienced a 43% miscarriage rate (9 miscarriages/21 pregnancies) compared with the control patients with fibroids who did not have surgery and who experienced a 56% miscarriage rate (5 miscarriages/9 pregnancies).[150] Thus, myomectomy for submucosal fibroids seems to lower the first-trimester miscarriage rate, but the outcomes are not significantly different ($\chi^2 = 0.41$, $P = .523$). Normally, randomized controlled trials are characterized as the highest level of evidence. However, the Cochrane review graded this study to have very low quality of evidence, in part because the sample size is so small and because different techniques (laparotomy and hysteroscopy) were used to perform the myomectomies.

Hysteroscopic myomectomy is recommended for submucosal fibroids that are 5 cm or less in diameter, although the procedure may necessitate additional steps if more than half of the fibroid is intramural.[8] A comprehensive review by Di Spiezio Sardo and colleagues[151] evaluated the numerous myomectomy techniques that may be considered, depending on the characteristics of the fibroids and the training of the surgeon, and discussed operative and postoperative complications. For women with RPL, complications that may affect future attempted pregnancies include the formation of intrauterine adhesions and the risk of uterine rupture during pregnancy.[151]

Nonhysteroscopic myomectomy may be considered in certain cases. A vaginal approach may be preferred if the fibroid penetrates the cervical canal.[8] If a submucosal fibroid is transmural, or if a hysteroscopic approach might damage too much of the endometrium, then an abdominal approach (eg, laparoscopy) might be used.[8] Several recent reviews have discussed in detail the advantages and disadvantages of the different types of nonhysteroscopic surgeries.[8,146]

Uterine artery embolization destroys fibroids by restricting their blood supply.[8,146] It is not recommended for patients with RPL, because it may cause amenorrhea and endometrial changes and was found to increase the risk of miscarriages compared with patients with fibroids who had not had treatment.[8,152]

Energy-based ablation uses energy sources such as radiofrequency-generated heat or magnetic resonance–guided ultrasonic waves to destroy fibroids; recent reviews have provided additional information about these procedures.[8,146]

Expectant management may be considered, particularly given the lack of definitive data in support of a specific treatment. The greatest problem with this approach is that women get older with each consecutive loss, and age increases not only the risk of miscarriage but also the likelihood of developing fibroids.[63,130,131]

- Submucosal fibroids increase rates of miscarriage, although the mechanism responsible for this is unknown.
- Fibroid development is polygenic and multifactorial. Estrogen, progesterone, growth factors, and other autocrine signaling molecules can promote fibroid growth.
- For women with early RPL who have submucosal fibroids, myomectomy should be considered if no other causes have been identified.

Polyps

Characteristics and classification

Polyps are benign growths of the endometrium, containing both glandular and stromal elements, including blood vessels. As described by Peterson and Novak,[153] polyps may be sessile, with a thick and plaquelike base or pedunculated, sometimes extending into or through the cervix. In their study, multiple polyps were found in 22% of the 616 uteri examined, and the size of any 1 polyp ranged from 0.3 to 12 cm. Polyps may have a functional endometrium, which responds to ovarian hormones in the manner of the surrounding endometrium, or may have an endometrium that is nonresponsive.[153]

Cause

Increased age and obesity are risk factors for polyps in premenopausal women.[154,155] Although there is no evidence of a heritable basis for polyps within families, polyps can show some characteristic chromosomal abnormalities. A cytogenetic study of 33 polyps found that 57% showed rearrangements in chromosomes 6 (6p21–22), 12 (12q13–15), and 7 (7q22).[156] These rearrangements are aberrations of the same chromosomal regions as those reported for fibroids, and all of these sites contain regulatory genes such as *HMG*.[113,156] Possibly, the same chromosomal anomalies in polyps and fibroids are a consequence of their common origin from invaginating cells of the embryonic coelomic epithelium.[156]

Like fibroids, polyps proliferate in response to estrogen and progesterone, growth factors, and other cytokines.[10,157] Increased aromatase activity within polyps may also contribute to growth through local production of estrogen.[158] Because polyps arise from endometrial tissue, which requires a complex balance of hormonal signals for its cyclical growth and degeneration, polyp growth is believed to be promoted by shifts in the relative expression of estrogen and progesterone receptors.[10,157] Also, data reviewed by Indraccolo and colleagues[157] suggest that polyp growth may be tied to cytokines that promote angiogenesis or to factors that inhibit normal apoptosis of the endometrium. Evidence in support of a specific mechanism is ambiguous, possibly because studies have not always accounted for differences in the expression of receptors and other proteins between the epithelium and the stroma of the polyps, or for differences in expression related to various stages of the menstrual cycle.[10]

Prevalence

A meta-analysis of studies that used SHG or hysteroscopy to diagnose polyps reported them in 2.4% of the patients with RPL (see **Table 5**D), making them the least common of the acquired uterine anomalies. In contrast, SHG examinations of asymptomatic premenopausal women (ie, women without abnormal uterine bleeding) found polyps in 7.6% (17/225) of women aged 20 years or older,[154] and in 10% (10/100) of women aged 30 years or older.[159] Because polyp prevalence increases with age,[154] this complicates comparisons among investigations that use patients of different ages.

First-trimester pregnancy loss

Several studies, including a randomized controlled trial, have linked endometrial polyps to infertility.[160] In contrast, the role of polyps in pregnancy loss has received little attention. Polyps are often lumped together with fibroids as contributors to miscarriage (eg, Devi Wold and colleagues[161]), and most studies of acquired uterine anomalies and RPL have reported them.[45,57,58,91] Clearly, there is a need to investigate the role that polyps might play in women with pregnancy loss.

Treatment options

A 2013 Cochrane systematic review of the effectiveness of polypectomy for infertile or subfertile women found only 1 randomized controlled trial, which did not report the impact of the surgery on miscarriage rate.[162] Two retrospective studies found no difference in first-trimester miscarriage rates between IVF patients who had received a polypectomy and those who had not; however, each investigation analyzed only 11 or fewer pregnancies per group.[163,164] As a result, these data were underpowered and less likely to reveal a statistically significant difference. If polyps are found in a workup for women with RPL and no other known cause, a polypectomy may be considered if the polyp is greater than 1 cm.[10,29] This size criterion is suggested because smaller polyps have been observed to regress in some patients.[165]

Methods of polyp removal reviewed by Salim and colleagues[10] include blind D&C, and also hysteroscopy with different techniques and tools for extracting the polyps. Given the risk of developing adhesions after D&C, and the reported ineffectiveness of D&C for removing polyps, one of the hysteroscopic resection techniques should be performed, based on the availability of equipment and training of the surgeon.[10]

- Polyp growth is affected by a balance of estrogen, progesterone, growth factors, and other autocrine signaling molecules, and factors that cause angiogenesis or inhibit apoptosis may affect polyp growth.
- Given the paucity of published data, there is a need for investigations concerning the role of polyps in first-trimester pregnancy loss, recurrent or otherwise.
- Hysteroscopic polypectomy may be considered for women with RPL if the polyp is large and no other causes have been found.

SUMMARY

Uterine anomalies are one of the most common factors associated with RPL. Congenital anomalies, such as bicornuate, unicornuate, didelphic, and septate uteri, most likely result from HOX mutations in the developing Müllerian duct. Of the acquired uterine anomalies, adhesions are typically formed after endometrial trauma, such as curettage, whereas fibroids and polyps are benign growths of the myometrium and endometrium, respectively. Many studies have explored the effects of uterine anomalies with respect to reproductive outcomes, but there are few randomized controlled trials, particularly for patients with RPL, and treatment methods lack strong supporting evidence. Nonetheless, metroplasty to correct a septate uterus and surgical removal of severe adhesions are recommended, and myomectomy of submucosal fibroids should be considered if no other causes have been identified.

REFERENCES

1. Sugiura-Ogasawara M, Suzuki S, Ozaki Y, et al. Frequency of recurrent spontaneous abortion and its influence on further marital relationship and illness: the Okazaki Cohort Study in Japan. J Obstet Gynaecol Res 2013;39:126–31.
2. Klock SC, Chang G, Hiley A, et al. Psychological distress among women with recurrent spontaneous abortion. Psychosomatics 1997;38:503–7.
3. Sugiura-Ogasawara M, Ozaki Y, Katano K, et al. Abnormal embryonic karyotype is the most frequent cause of recurrent miscarriage. Hum Reprod 2012;27:2297–303.
4. Jauniaux E, Farquharson RG, Christiansen OB, et al. Evidence-based guidelines for the investigation and medical treatment of recurrent miscarriage. Hum Reprod 2006;21:2216–22.

5. Jaslow CR, Carney JL, Kutteh WH. Diagnostic factors identified in 1020 women with two versus three or more recurrent pregnancy losses. Fertil Steril 2010;93: 1234–43.

6. Chan YY, Jayaprakasan K, Zamora J, et al. The prevalence of congenital uterine anomalies in unselected and high-risk populations: a systematic review. Hum Reprod Update 2011;17:761–71.

7. Saravelos SH, Cocksedge KA, Li TC. Prevalence and diagnosis of congenital uterine anomalies in women with reproductive failure: a critical appraisal. Hum Reprod Update 2008;14:415–29.

8. American Association of Gynecologic Laparoscopists: Advancing Minimally Invasive Gynecology Worldwide. AAGL practice report: practice guidelines for the diagnosis and management of submucous leiomyomas. J Minim Invasive Gynecol 2012;19:152–71.

9. AAGL Advancing Minimally Invasive Gynecology Worldwide. AAGL practice report: practice guidelines for management of intrauterine synechiae. J Minim Invasive Gynecol 2010;17:1–7.

10. Salim S, Won H, Nesbitt-Hawes E, et al. Diagnosis and management of endometrial polyps: a critical review of the literature. J Minim Invasive Gynecol 2011;18: 569–81.

11. Salim R, Lee C, Davies A, et al. A comparative study of three-dimensional saline infusion sonohysterography and diagnostic hysteroscopy for the classification of submucous fibroids. Hum Reprod 2005;20:253–7.

12. Hashimoto R. Development of the human Müllerian duct in the sexually undifferentiated stage. Anat Rec A Discov Mol Cell Evol Biol 2003;272:514–9.

13. Lee DM, Osathanondh R, Yeh J. Localization of Bcl-2 in the human fetal Müllerian tract. Fertil Steril 1998;70:135–40.

14. Toaff ME, Lev-Toaff AS, Toaff R. Communicating uteri: review and classification with introduction of two previously unreported types. Fertil Steril 1984;41: 661–79.

15. Guioli S, Sekido R, Lovell-Badge R. The origin of the Müllerian duct in chick and mouse. Dev Biol 2007;302:389–98.

16. Orvis GD, Behringer RR. Cellular mechanisms of Müllerian duct formation in the mouse. Dev Biol 2007;306:493–504.

17. Masse J, Watrin T, Laurent A, et al. The developing female genital tract: from genetics to epigenetics. Int J Dev Biol 2009;53:411–24.

18. Kurita T, Cooke PS, Cunha GR. Epithelial-stromal tissue interaction in paramesonephric (Müllerian) epithelial differentiation. Dev Biol 2001;240:194–211.

19. Kitajewski J, Sassoon D. The emergence of molecular gynecology: homeobox and Wnt genes in the female reproductive tract. Bioessays 2000;22:902–10.

20. Miller C, Sassoon DA. Wnt-7a maintains appropriate uterine patterning during the development of the mouse female reproductive tract. Development 1998; 125:3201–11.

21. Taylor HS, Vanden Heuvel GB, Igarashi P. A conserved Hox axis in the mouse and human female reproductive system: late establishment and persistent adult expression of the Hoxa cluster genes. Biol Reprod 1997;57:1338–45.

22. Cunha GR, Young P, Brody JR. Role of uterine epithelium in the development of myometrial smooth muscle cells. Biol Reprod 1989;40:861–71.

23. AFS. The American Fertility Society classifications of adnexal adhesions, distal tubal occlusion, tubal occlusion secondary to tubal ligation, tubal pregnancies, Müllerian anomalies and intrauterine adhesions. Fertil Steril 1988;49: 944–55.

24. Kara T, Acu B, Beyhan M, et al. MRI in the diagnosis of Mayer-Rokitansky-Kuster-Hauser syndrome. Diagn Interv Radiol 2013;19:227–32.
25. Acien P, Acien MI. The history of female genital tract malformation classifications and proposal of an updated system. Hum Reprod Update 2011;17:693–705.
26. Reichman D, Laufer MR, Robinson BK. Pregnancy outcomes in unicornuate uteri: a review. Fertil Steril 2009;91:1886–94.
27. Nahum GG. Uterine anomalies. How common are they, and what is their distribution among subtypes? J Reprod Med 1998;43:877–87.
28. Nahum GG, Stanislaw H, McMahon C. Preventing ectopic pregnancies: how often does transperitoneal transmigration of sperm occur in effecting human pregnancy? BJOG 2004;111:706–14.
29. Taylor E, Gomel V. The uterus and fertility. Fertil Steril 2008;89:1–16.
30. Troiano RN, McCarthy SM. Müllerian duct anomalies: imaging and clinical issues. Radiology 2004;233:19–34.
31. Homer HA, Li TC, Cooke ID. The septate uterus: a review of management and reproductive outcome. Fertil Steril 2000;73:1–14.
32. Pellerito JS, McCarthy SM, Doyle MB, et al. Diagnosis of uterine anomalies: relative accuracy of MR imaging, endovaginal sonography, and hysterosalpingography. Radiology 1992;183:795–800.
33. Reuter KL, Daly DC, Cohen SM. Septate versus bicornuate uteri: errors in imaging diagnosis. Radiology 1989;172:749–52.
34. Reichman DE, Laufer MR. Congenital uterine anomalies affecting reproduction. Best Pract Res Clin Obstet Gynaecol 2010;24:193–208.
35. Grimbizis GF, Campo R. Clinical approach for the classification of congenital uterine malformations. Gynecol Surg 2012;9:119–29.
36. Sparac V, Kupesic S, Ilijas M, et al. Histologic architecture and vascularization of hysteroscopically excised intrauterine septa. J Am Assoc Gynecol Laparosc 2001;8:111–6.
37. Candiani GB, Fedele L, Zamberletti D, et al. Endometrial patterns in malformed uteri. Acta Eur Fertil 1983;14:311–8.
38. Dabirashrafi H, Bahadori M, Mohammad K, et al. Septate uterus: new idea on the histologic features of the septum in this abnormal uterus. Am J Obstet Gynecol 1995;172:105–7.
39. Makino T, Umeuchi M, Nakada K, et al. Incidence of congenital uterine anomalies in repeated reproductive wastage and prognosis for pregnancy after metroplasty. Int J Fertil 1992;37:167–70.
40. Woelfer B, Salim R, Banerjee S, et al. Reproductive outcomes in women with congenital uterine anomalies detected by three-dimensional ultrasound screening. Obstet Gynecol 2001;98:1099–103.
41. Sørensen SS, Trauelsen AG. Obstetric implications of minor Müllerian anomalies in oligomenorrheic women. Am J Obstet Gynecol 1987;156:1112–8.
42. Valli E, Zupi E, Marconi D, et al. Hysteroscopic findings in 344 women with recurrent spontaneous abortion. J Am Assoc Gynecol Laparosc 2001;8:398–401.
43. Lin PC, Bhatnagar KP, Nettleton GS, et al. Female genital anomalies affecting reproduction. Fertil Steril 2002;78:899–915.
44. Ghi T, Casadio P, Kuleva M, et al. Accuracy of three-dimensional ultrasound in diagnosis and classification of congenital uterine anomalies. Fertil Steril 2009; 92:808–13.
45. Jaslow CR, Kutteh WH. Effect of prior birth and miscarriage frequency on the prevalence of acquired and congenital uterine anomalies in women with recurrent miscarriage: a cross-sectional study. Fertil Steril 2013;99:1916–22.e1.

46. Salim R, Regan L, Woelfer B, et al. A comparative study of the morphology of congenital uterine anomalies in women with and without a history of recurrent first trimester miscarriage. Hum Reprod 2003;18:162–6.
47. Stephenson MD. Frequency of factors associated with habitual abortion in 197 couples. Fertil Steril 1996;66:24–9.
48. Kaufman RH, Binder GL, Gray PM Jr, et al. Upper genital tract changes associated with exposure in utero to diethylstilbestrol. Am J Obstet Gynecol 1977;128: 51–9.
49. Ma L, Benson GV, Lim H, et al. Abdominal B (AbdB) Hoxa genes: regulation in adult uterus by estrogen and progesterone and repression in Müllerian duct by the synthetic estrogen diethylstilbestrol (DES). Dev Biol 1998;197:141–54.
50. Suzuki A, Urushitani H, Sato T, et al. Gene expression change in the Müllerian duct of the mouse fetus exposed to diethylstilbestrol in utero. Exp Biol Med (Maywood) 2007;232:503–14.
51. Block K, Kardana A, Igarashi P, et al. In utero diethylstilbestrol (DES) exposure alters Hox gene expression in the developing Müllerian system. FASEB J 2000; 14:1101–8.
52. Goodman FR, Bacchelli C, Brady AF, et al. Novel HOXA13 mutations and the phenotypic spectrum of hand-foot-genital syndrome. Am J Hum Genet 2000; 67:197–202.
53. Cheng Z, Zhu Y, Su D, et al. A novel mutation of HOXA10 in a Chinese woman with a Müllerian duct anomaly. Hum Reprod 2011;26:3197–201.
54. Hammoud AO, Gibson M, Peterson CM, et al. Quantification of the familial contribution to Müllerian anomalies. Obstet Gynecol 2008;111:378–84.
55. Elias S, Simpson JL, Carson SA, et al. Genetics studies in incomplete Müllerian fusion. Obstet Gynecol 1984;63:276–9.
56. Souza CA, Schmitz C, Genro VK, et al. Office hysteroscopy study in consecutive miscarriage patients. Rev Assoc Med Bras 2011;57:397–401.
57. Weiss A, Shalev E, Romano S. Hysteroscopy may be justified after two miscarriages. Hum Reprod 2005;20:2628–31.
58. Bohlmann MK, von Wolff M, Luedders DW, et al. Hysteroscopic findings in women with two and with more than two first-trimester miscarriages are not significantly different. Reprod Biomed Online 2010;21:230–6.
59. Bax L. MIX 2.0. Professional software for meta-analysis in Excel. Version (2.0.1.4). 2011. Available at: http://www.meta-analysis-made-easy.com. Accessed May 24, 2012.
60. Tulppala M, Palosuo T, Ramsay T, et al. A prospective study of 63 couples with a history of recurrent spontaneous abortion: contributing factors and outcome of subsequent pregnancies. Hum Reprod 1993;8:764–70.
61. Hanley JA, Lippman-Hand A. If nothing goes wrong, is everything all right? Interpreting zero numerators. JAMA 1983;249:1743–5.
62. Warburton D, Fraser FC. Spontaneous abortion risks in man: data from reproductive histories collected in a medical genetics unit. Am J Hum Genet 1964;16:1–25.
63. Nybo Andersen AM, Wohlfahrt J, Christens P, et al. Maternal age and fetal loss: population based register linkage study. BMJ 2000;320:1708–12.
64. Chan YY, Jayaprakasan K, Tan A, et al. Reproductive outcomes in women with congenital uterine anomalies: a systematic review. Ultrasound Obstet Gynecol 2011;38:371–82.
65. Jayaprakasan K, Chan YY, Sur S, et al. Prevalence of uterine anomalies and their impact on early pregnancy in women conceiving after assisted reproduction treatment. Ultrasound Obstet Gynecol 2011;37:727–32.

66. Raga F, Bauset C, Remohi J, et al. Reproductive impact of congenital Müllerian anomalies. Hum Reprod 1997;12:2277–81.
67. Zlopasa G, Skrablin S, Kalafatic D, et al. Uterine anomalies and pregnancy outcome following resectoscope metroplasty. Int J Gynaecol Obstet 2007;98: 129–33.
68. Saravelos SH, Cocksedge KA, Li TC. The pattern of pregnancy loss in women with congenital uterine anomalies and recurrent miscarriage. Reprod Biomed Online 2010;20:416–22.
69. Fedele L, Dorta M, Brioschi D, et al. Pregnancies in septate uteri: outcome in relation to site of uterine implantation as determined by sonography. AJR Am J Roentgenol 1989;152:781–4.
70. Fedele L, Bianchi S, Marchini M, et al. Ultrastructural aspects of endometrium in infertile women with septate uterus. Fertil Steril 1996;65:750–2.
71. Leible S, Cumsille F, Walton R, et al. Discordant uterine artery velocity waveforms as a predictor of subsequent miscarriage in early viable pregnancies. Am J Obstet Gynecol 1998;179:1587–93.
72. Leible S, Munoz H, Walton R, et al. Uterine artery blood flow velocity waveforms in pregnant women with Müllerian duct anomaly: a biologic model for uteroplacental insufficiency. Am J Obstet Gynecol 1998;178:1048–53.
73. Burchell RC, Creed F, Rasoulpour M, et al. Vascular anatomy of the human uterus and pregnancy wastage. Br J Obstet Gynaecol 1978;85:698–706.
74. Andrews MC, Jones HW Jr. Impaired reproductive performance of the unicornuate uterus: intrauterine growth retardation, infertility, and recurrent abortion in five cases. Am J Obstet Gynecol 1982;144:173–6.
75. Alborzi S, Asadi N, Zolghadri J, et al. Laparoscopic metroplasty in bicornuate and didelphic uteri. Fertil Steril 2009;92:352–5.
76. Brucker SY, Rall K, Campo R, et al. Treatment of congenital malformations. Semin Reprod Med 2011;29:101–12.
77. Rackow BW, Arici A. Reproductive performance of women with Müllerian anomalies. Curr Opin Obstet Gynecol 2007;19:229–37.
78. Musich JR, Behrman SJ. Obstetric outcome before and after metroplasty in women with uterine anomalies. Obstet Gynecol 1978;52:63–6.
79. Kowalik CR, Goddijn M, Emanuel MH, et al. Metroplasty versus expectant management for women with recurrent miscarriage and a septate uterus. Cochrane Database Syst Rev 2011;(6):CD008576.
80. Valle RF, Ekpo GE. Hysteroscopic metroplasty for the septate uterus: review and meta-analysis. J Minim Invasive Gynecol 2013;20:22–42.
81. Grimbizis GF, Camus M, Tarlatzis BC, et al. Clinical implications of uterine malformations and hysteroscopic treatment results. Hum Reprod Update 2001;7: 161–74.
82. Daly DC, Maier D, Soto-Albors C. Hysteroscopic metroplasty: six years' experience. Obstet Gynecol 1989;73:201–5.
83. Lin PC. Reproductive outcomes in women with uterine anomalies. J Womens Health (Larchmt) 2004;13:33–9.
84. Ban-Frangez H, Tomazevic T, Virant-Klun I, et al. The outcome of singleton pregnancies after IVF/ICSI in women before and after hysteroscopic resection of a uterine septum compared to normal controls. Eur J Obstet Gynecol Reprod Biol 2009;146:184–7.
85. Gergolet M, Campo R, Verdenik I, et al. No clinical relevance of the height of fundal indentation in subseptate or arcuate uterus: a prospective study. Reprod Biomed Online 2012;24:576–82.

86. Giacomucci E, Bellavia E, Sandri F, et al. Term delivery rate after hysteroscopic metroplasty in patients with recurrent spontaneous abortion and T-shaped, arcuate and septate uterus. Gynecol Obstet Invest 2011;71:183–8.
87. Golan A, Langer R, Wexler S, et al. Cervical cerclage–its role in the pregnant anomalous uterus. Int J Fertil 1990;35:164–70.
88. Ventolini G, Zhang M, Gruber J. Hysteroscopy in the evaluation of patients with recurrent pregnancy loss: a cohort study in a primary care population. Surg Endosc 2004;18:1782–4.
89. Dendrinos S, Grigoriou O, Sakkas EG, et al. Hysteroscopy in the evaluation of habitual abortions. Eur J Contracept Reprod Health Care 2008;13:198–200.
90. Guimarães Filho HA, Mattar R, Pires CR, et al. Prevalence of uterine defects in habitual abortion patients attended on at a university health service in Brazil. Arch Gynecol Obstet 2006;274:345–8.
91. Cogendez E, Dolgun ZN, Sanverdi I, et al. Post-abortion hysteroscopy: a method for early diagnosis of congenital and acquired intrauterine causes of abortions. Eur J Obstet Gynecol Reprod Biol 2011;156:101–4.
92. Raziel A, Arieli S, Bukovsky I, et al. Investigation of the uterine cavity in recurrent aborters. Fertil Steril 1994;62:1080–2.
93. Coulam CB. Epidemiology of recurrent spontaneous abortion. Am J Reprod Immunol 1991;26:23–7.
94. March CM. Management of Asherman's syndrome. Reprod Biomed Online 2011;23:63–76.
95. Yu D, Wong YM, Cheong Y, et al. Asherman syndrome–one century later. Fertil Steril 2008;89:759–79.
96. Foix A, Bruno RO, Davison T, et al. The pathology of postcurettage intrauterine adhesions. Am J Obstet Gynecol 1966;96:1027–33.
97. Valle RF, Sciarra JJ. Intrauterine adhesions: hysteroscopic diagnosis, classification, treatment, and reproductive outcome. Am J Obstet Gynecol 1988;158:1459–70.
98. Al-Inany H. Intrauterine adhesions. An update. Acta Obstet Gynecol Scand 2001;80:986–93.
99. Schenker JG, Margalioth EJ. Intrauterine adhesions: an updated appraisal. Fertil Steril 1982;37:593–610.
100. Deans R, Abbott J. Review of intrauterine adhesions. J Minim Invasive Gynecol 2010;17:555–69.
101. Friedler S, Margalioth EJ, Kafka I, et al. Incidence of post-abortion intra-uterine adhesions evaluated by hysteroscopy–a prospective study. Hum Reprod 1993; 8:442–4.
102. Westendorp IC, Ankum WM, Mol BW, et al. Prevalence of Asherman's syndrome after secondary removal of placental remnants or a repeat curettage for incomplete abortion. Hum Reprod 1998;13:3347–50.
103. Romer T. Post-abortion-hysteroscopy–a method for early diagnosis of congenital and acquired intrauterine causes of abortions. Eur J Obstet Gynecol Reprod Biol 1994;57:171–3.
104. Li TC, Iqbal T, Anstie B, et al. An analysis of the pattern of pregnancy loss in women with recurrent miscarriage. Fertil Steril 2002;78:1100–6.
105. Cooper JM, Houck RM, Rigberg HS. The incidence of intrauterine abnormalities found at hysteroscopy in patients undergoing elective hysteroscopic sterilization. J Reprod Med 1983;28:659–61.
106. Fatemi HM, Kasius JC, Timmermans A, et al. Prevalence of unsuspected uterine cavity abnormalities diagnosed by office hysteroscopy prior to in vitro fertilization. Hum Reprod 2010;25:1959–65.

107. Taylor PJ, Cumming DC, Hill PJ. Significance of intrauterine adhesions detected hysteroscopically in eumenorrheic infertile women and role of antecedent curettage in their formation. Am J Obstet Gynecol 1981;139:239–42.
108. Polishuk WZ, Sadovsky E. A syndrome of recurrent intrauterine adhesions. Am J Obstet Gynecol 1975;123:151–8.
109. Yaffe H, Ron M, Polishuk WZ. Amenorrhea, hypomenorrhea, and uterine fibrosis. Am J Obstet Gynecol 1978;130:599–601.
110. Polishuk WZ, Siew FP, Gordon R, et al. Vascular changes in traumatic amenorrhea and hypomenorrhea. Int J Fertil 1977;22:189–92.
111. Yu D, Li TC, Xia E, et al. Factors affecting reproductive outcome of hysteroscopic adhesiolysis for Asherman's syndrome. Fertil Steril 2008;89:715–22.
112. Ciarmela P, Islam MS, Reis FM, et al. Growth factors and myometrium: biological effects in uterine fibroid and possible clinical implications. Hum Reprod Update 2011;17:772–90.
113. Flake GP, Andersen J, Dixon D. Etiology and pathogenesis of uterine leiomyomas: a review. Environ Health Perspect 2003;111:1037–54.
114. Richards PA, Richards PD, Tiltman AJ. The ultrastructure of fibromyomatous myometrium and its relationship to infertility. Hum Reprod Update 1998;4: 520–5.
115. Malik M, Norian J, McCarthy-Keith D, et al. Why leiomyomas are called fibroids: the central role of extracellular matrix in symptomatic women. Semin Reprod Med 2010;28:169–79.
116. Moore AB, Yu L, Swartz CD, et al. Human uterine leiomyoma-derived fibroblasts stimulate uterine leiomyoma cell proliferation and collagen type I production, and activate RTKs and TGF beta receptor signaling in coculture. Cell Commun Signal 2010;8:10.
117. Islam MS, Protic O, Stortoni P, et al. Complex networks of multiple factors in the pathogenesis of uterine leiomyoma. Fertil Steril 2013;100(1):178–93.
118. Eiletz J, Genz T, Pollow K, et al. Sex steroid levels in serum, myometrium, and fibromyomata in correlation with cytoplasmic receptors and 17 beta-HSD activity in different age-groups and phases of the menstrual cycle. Arch Gynecol 1980;229:13–28.
119. Bakas P, Liapis A, Vlahopoulos S, et al. Estrogen receptor alpha and beta in uterine fibroids: a basis for altered estrogen responsiveness. Fertil Steril 2008; 90:1878–85.
120. Lv J, Zhu X, Dong K, et al. Reduced expression of 14-3-3 gamma in uterine leiomyoma as identified by proteomics. Fertil Steril 2008;90:1892–8.
121. Suo G, Jiang Y, Cowan B, et al. Platelet-derived growth factor C is upregulated in human uterine fibroids and regulates uterine smooth muscle cell growth. Biol Reprod 2009;81:749–58.
122. Murase E, Siegelman ES, Outwater EK, et al. Uterine leiomyomas: histopathologic features, MR imaging findings, differential diagnosis, and treatment. Radiographics 1999;19:1179–97.
123. Bajekal N, Li TC. Fibroids, infertility and pregnancy wastage. Hum Reprod Update 2000;6:614–20.
124. Ligon AH, Morton CC. Genetics of uterine leiomyomata. Genes Chromosomes Cancer 2000;28:235–45.
125. Brosens I, Deprest J, Dal Cin P, et al. Clinical significance of cytogenetic abnormalities in uterine myomas. Fertil Steril 1998;69:232–5.
126. Rein MS, Powell WL, Walters FC, et al. Cytogenetic abnormalities in uterine myomas are associated with myoma size. Mol Hum Reprod 1998;4:83–6.

127. Asada H, Yamagata Y, Taketani T, et al. Potential link between estrogen receptor-alpha gene hypomethylation and uterine fibroid formation. Mol Hum Reprod 2008;14:539–45.
128. Linder D, Gartler SM. Glucose-6-phosphate dehydrogenase mosaicism: utilization as a cell marker in the study of leiomyomas. Science 1965;150:67–9.
129. Vikhlyaeva EM, Khodzhaeva ZS, Fantschenko ND. Familial predisposition to uterine leiomyomas. Int J Gynaecol Obstet 1995;51:127–31.
130. Baird DD, Dunson DB, Hill MC, et al. High cumulative incidence of uterine leiomyoma in black and white women: ultrasound evidence. Am J Obstet Gynecol 2003;188:100–7.
131. Marshall LM, Spiegelman D, Barbieri RL, et al. Variation in the incidence of uterine leiomyoma among premenopausal women by age and race. Obstet Gynecol 1997;90:967–73.
132. Eggert SL, Huyck KL, Somasundaram P, et al. Genome-wide linkage and association analyses implicate FASN in predisposition to uterine leiomyomata. Am J Hum Genet 2012;91:621–8.
133. Hodge JC, T Cuenco K, Huyck KL, et al. Uterine leiomyomata and decreased height: a common HMGA2 predisposition allele. Hum Genet 2009;125:257–63.
134. Cramer SF, Patel A. The frequency of uterine leiomyomas. Am J Clin Pathol 1990;94:435–8.
135. Borgfeldt C, Andolf E. Transvaginal ultrasonographic findings in the uterus and the endometrium: low prevalence of leiomyoma in a random sample of women age 25-40 years. Acta Obstet Gynecol Scand 2000;79:202–7.
136. Laughlin SK, Baird DD, Savitz DA, et al. Prevalence of uterine leiomyomas in the first trimester of pregnancy: an ultrasound-screening study. Obstet Gynecol 2009;113:630–5.
137. Marsh EE, Ekpo GE, Cardozo ER, et al. Racial differences in fibroid prevalence and ultrasound findings in asymptomatic young women (18-30 years old): a pilot study. Fertil Steril 2013;99:1951–7.
138. Klatsky PC, Tran ND, Caughey AB, et al. Fibroids and reproductive outcomes: a systematic literature review from conception to delivery. Am J Obstet Gynecol 2008;198:357–66.
139. Pritts EA, Parker WH, Olive DL. Fibroids and infertility: an updated systematic review of the evidence. Fertil Steril 2009;91:1215–23.
140. Sunkara SK, Khairy M, El-Toukhy T, et al. The effect of intramural fibroids without uterine cavity involvement on the outcome of IVF treatment: a systematic review and meta-analysis. Hum Reprod 2010;25:418–29.
141. Saravelos SH, Yan J, Rehmani H, et al. The prevalence and impact of fibroids and their treatment on the outcome of pregnancy in women with recurrent miscarriage. Hum Reprod 2011;26:3274–9.
142. Deligdish L, Loewenthal M. Endometrial changes associated with myomata of the uterus. J Clin Pathol 1970;23:676–80.
143. Sinclair DC, Mastroyannis A, Taylor HS. Leiomyoma simultaneously impair endometrial BMP-2-mediated decidualization and anticoagulant expression through secretion of TGF-beta3. J Clin Endocrinol Metab 2011;96:412–21.
144. Makker A, Goel MM. Uterine leiomyomas: effects on architectural, cellular, and molecular determinants of endometrial receptivity. Reprod Sci 2013;20:631–8.
145. Miura S, Khan KN, Kitajima M, et al. Differential infiltration of macrophages and prostaglandin production by different uterine leiomyomas. Hum Reprod 2006;21:2545–54.

146. Guo XC, Segars JH. The impact and management of fibroids for fertility: an evidence-based approach. Obstet Gynecol Clin North Am 2012;39:521–33.
147. Roy KK, Singla S, Baruah J, et al. Reproductive outcome following hysteroscopic myomectomy in patients with infertility and recurrent abortions. Arch Gynecol Obstet 2010;282:553–60.
148. Shokeir TA. Hysteroscopic management in submucous fibroids to improve fertility. Arch Gynecol Obstet 2005;273:50–4.
149. Metwally M, Cheong YC, Horne AW. Surgical treatment of fibroids for subfertility. Cochrane Database Syst Rev 2012;(11):CD003857.
150. Casini ML, Rossi F, Agostini R, et al. Effects of the position of fibroids on fertility. Gynecol Endocrinol 2006;22:106–9.
151. Di Spiezio Sardo A, Mazzon I, Bramante S, et al. Hysteroscopic myomectomy: a comprehensive review of surgical techniques. Hum Reprod Update 2008;14:101–19.
152. Homer H, Saridogan E. Uterine artery embolization for fibroids is associated with an increased risk of miscarriage. Fertil Steril 2010;94:324–30.
153. Peterson WF, Novak ER. Endometrial polyps. Obstet Gynecol 1956;8:40–9.
154. Dreisler E, Stampe Sorensen S, Ibsen PH, et al. Prevalence of endometrial polyps and abnormal uterine bleeding in a Danish population aged 20-74 years. Ultrasound Obstet Gynecol 2009;33:102–8.
155. Onalan R, Onalan G, Tonguc E, et al. Body mass index is an independent risk factor for the development of endometrial polyps in patients undergoing in vitro fertilization. Fertil Steril 2009;91:1056–60.
156. Dal Cin P, Vanni R, Marras S, et al. Four cytogenetic subgroups can be identified in endometrial polyps. Cancer Res 1995;55:1565–8.
157. Indraccolo U, Di Iorio R, Matteo M, et al. The pathogenesis of endometrial polyps: a systematic semi-quantitative review. Eur J Gynaecol Oncol 2013;34:5–22.
158. Maia H Jr, Pimentel K, Silva TM, et al. Aromatase and cyclooxygenase-2 expression in endometrial polyps during the menstrual cycle. Gynecol Endocrinol 2006;22:219–24.
159. Clevenger-Hoeft M, Syrop CH, Stovall DW, et al. Sonohysterography in premenopausal women with and without abnormal bleeding. Obstet Gynecol 1999;94:516–20.
160. Perez-Medina T, Bajo-Arenas J, Salazar F, et al. Endometrial polyps and their implication in the pregnancy rates of patients undergoing intrauterine insemination: a prospective, randomized study. Hum Reprod 2005;20:1632–5.
161. Devi Wold AS, Pham N, Arici A. Anatomic factors in recurrent pregnancy loss. Semin Reprod Med 2006;24:25–32.
162. Bosteels J, Kasius J, Weyers S, et al. Hysteroscopy for treating subfertility associated with suspected major uterine cavity abnormalities. Cochrane Database Syst Rev 2013;(1):CD009461.
163. Check JH, Bostick-Smith CA, Choe JK, et al. Matched controlled study to evaluate the effect of endometrial polyps on pregnancy and implantation rates following in vitro fertilization-embryo transfer (IVF-ET). Clin Exp Obstet Gynecol 2011;38:206–8.
164. Lass A, Williams G, Abusheikha N, et al. The effect of endometrial polyps on outcomes of in vitro fertilization (IVF) cycles. J Assist Reprod Genet 1999;16:410–5.
165. Lieng M, Istre O, Sandvik L, et al. Prevalence, 1-year regression rate, and clinical significance of asymptomatic endometrial polyps: cross-sectional study. J Minim Invasive Gynecol 2009;16:465–71.

Mid-Trimester Pregnancy Loss

Kelly M. McNamee, MBChB[a],*, Feroza Dawood, MBChB, MRCOG, MD[a],
Roy G. Farquharson, MD, FRCOG[b]

KEYWORDS

- Mid-trimester loss • Late pregnancy loss • Recurrent miscarriage
- Miscarriage investigations • Antiphospholipid syndrome • Bacterial vaginosis
- Cerclage

KEY POINTS

- Women with mid-trimester pregnancy loss (MTL) represent a heterogeneous group, with widely varying presentations and origins.
- An implemented protocol with standardized investigations is essential to identify any potential cause for an MTL.
- Consideration for transabdominal cerclage requires appropriate patient selection.
- An MTL may have more than one cause; the presence of dual or even triple pathology increases the risk of a further MTL or preterm delivery dramatically.
- Well-designed trials to study MTL are required to establish robust evidence-based practice and improve the treatment and care clinicians can provide.

INTRODUCTION

Mid-trimester loss (MTL) is defined as a pregnancy loss between 12 and 24 weeks' gestation.[1] The true incidence of this complication is difficult to ascertain, because no accurate data collection has been published.[2] It is estimated to affect 2% to 3% of recognized pregnancies.[3] MTL has often been classified together with first trimester losses or omitted altogether. An overlap also exists among MTL, preterm delivery (PTD), and preterm prelabor rupture of membranes (PPROM), and these conditions may often be a continuum of associated factors. The distinction between MTL and PTD is defined as the gestation of fetal viability (currently 24 weeks' gestation); both complications are known to have a similar origin.[4]

A dearth of knowledge exists regarding the optimal treatment and investigations for a distinct MTL cohort. Women who have an MTL represent a heterogeneous group, displaying widely varying presentations and origins.[2] Causative factors include

Funding Sources: None.
Conflicts of Interest: None.
[a] Department of Obstetrics, Liverpool Women's Hospital, Crown Street, Liverpool L8 7SS, UK;
[b] Department of Gynaecology, Liverpool Women's Hospital, Crown Street, Liverpool L8 7SS, UK
* Corresponding author.
E-mail address: kellymcnamee@doctors.org.uk

antiphospholipid syndrome (APS), cervical weakness, infection, placental insufficiency, and congenital uterine anomalies (CUAs). Despite this, the cause remains unknown in 50% to 60% of women.[1–3,5] An important consideration is that an MTL may have more than one cause. The presence of dual or even triple pathology dramatically increases the risk of a further MTL or PTD.

An implemented protocol with standardized investigations is essential to identify any potential cause for an MTL. Classifying pathology is important for determining future pregnancy management, especially in the presence of repeated MTL.

SCREENING PROTOCOL

When investigating a woman with a history of an MTL, a thorough objective approach is required. An accurate clinical event history can often expose a potential cause (**Table 1**). A detailed family history can identify hereditary factors, such as thrombophilia or chromosomal translocation, thus guiding appropriate evaluation. Complex maternal illnesses, such as poorly controlled diabetes, uncontrolled hypertension, and thrombophilia, have been known to cause MTL. Poorly controlled thyroid disease is also associated with MTL and PTD; however, if the maternal disease has contributed to a pregnancy complication, confirmation should be sought as evidence (ie, placental pathology).[5] A sudden asymptomatic intrauterine death can be associated with APS, whereas cervical weakness classically presents as silent cervical dilatation with evidence of fetal heart activity. Infection can present as spontaneous rupture of membranes with a closed cervix.[2]

A clinical event picture can be mixed and difficult to interpret. Occasionally, women with more than one MTL can describe very different histories emphasizing the possibility of dual/triple pathology. Differing causal factors can predominate at different gestations in different pregnancies within the same individual.[2] Although a local investigative audit showed the distribution of pathology, it may not be truly representative of all MTLs because of referral bias (**Fig. 1**).

After a detailed history, a series of investigations should be performed (**Fig. 2**). Diagnosis of APS can be complex and is usually a combination of clinical manifestation and presence of lupus anticoagulant and/or anticardiolipin antibodies.[6] With a history of MTL, a high vaginal swab (HVS) can diagnose/exclude possible infection. A repeated HVS is recommended in the first trimester of a subsequent pregnancy to exclude bacterial vaginosis (BV), the presence of which may fluctuate over time. The Nugent criteria are used because they include an intermediate-flora classification characterized by abnormal genital-tract colonization that may be a transition stage on the way to full-fledged BV.[7] The cervix may be evaluated with a transvaginal ultrasound to measure cervical length and with hysteroscopy, but assessment also requires a convincing history. CUAs can also be diagnosed through ultrasound (3-dimensional if facilities allow) and/or hysteroscopy.

Table 1
Clinical history sequence

Event vs Factor	Cervix	Liquor Present on Vaginal Speculum Examination	Fetal Heart Activity
Cervical weakness	Open	Absent until expulsion of sac	Present
Thrombophilia/APS	Closed	Absent	Absent
Bacterial vaginosis	Closed	Present	?Present until sac expulsion

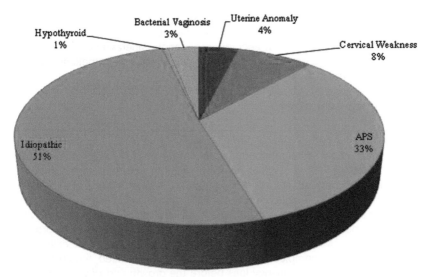

Fig. 1. Distribution of cause in 351 consecutive cases of MTL at Liverpool Women's Hospital.

Whether a previous MTL was a consequence of a chromosomal abnormality or fetal anomaly is advantageous to determine. Previous amniocentesis or postmortem results can potentially eliminate causative pathology. Increasing consensus is favoring full cytogenetic testing with array comparative genomic hybridization and fluorescent

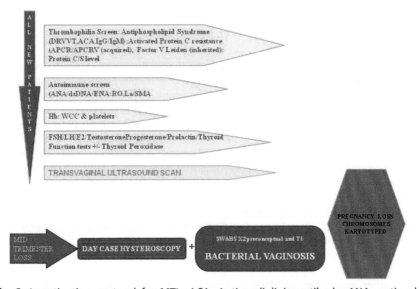

Fig. 2. Investigation protocol for MTL. ACA, Anti-cardiolipin antibody; ANA, antinuclear antibodies; DRVVT, Dilute Russell's viper venom time; dsDNA, double stranded Deoxyribonucleic acid; E2, Oestradiol; ENA, Extractable nuclear antigens; FSH, Follicular stimulating hormone; Hb, Haemoglobin; IgG, Immunoglobulin G; IgM, Immunoglobulin M; La, anti-La antibodies; LH, Luteinising hormone; RO, anti-Ro antibodies; SMA, Anti-Smith antibodies; WCC, White cell count. (*Adapted from* Farquharson RG. Late pregnancy loss. In: Farquharson RG, Stephenson MD, editors. Early pregnancy. Cambridge: Cambridge University Press; 2010. p. 277–86; with permission.)

in situ hybridization for all women who have experienced pregnancy losses. Debate exists as to whether the success or failure of a treatment in a previous pregnancy loss can ever be defined without accurate cytogenetic analysis. The chromosomal analysis of a miscarriage can be an informative diagnostic tool for patient counseling and subsequent pregnancy management.[8]

MTL–ASSOCIATED PATHOLOGY
APS

APS is associated with miscarriage in any trimester. It was first described in the early 1980s as a unique form of autoantibody-induced thrombophilia associated with pregnancy complications. The antibodies involved promote activation of the endothelial cells, monocytes, and platelets. As a consequence, tissue factor and thromboxane A2 is overproduced.[9] The most common obstetric manifestation is fetal loss; however, other features include preeclampsia and placental insufficiency, prompting delivery.[10] The hypothesis behind APS and pregnancy loss is the encouragement of a prothrombotic environment. Microthrombi are common in the placental vasculature and decidua in pregnancy samples from patients who experienced recurrent miscarriages.[11] APS can cause pregnancy loss before the growth and development of the placental vasculature. Inflammation is a significant component of APS pathogenesis, as demonstrated in recent mice studies showing a pivotal role of complement activation in thrombosis and fetal loss induced by antiphospholipid antibodies.[12] Although existing literature suggests that women with APS are more likely to experience a fetal loss in the first trimester,[13] convincing evidence shows that pregnancy complications are most prevalent in late pregnancy,[14] with one study reporting APS in 42% of a cohort with a history of MTL.[15]

TREATMENT

Guidelines are in place for the treatment of positively diagnosed APS with thromboprophylactic medication.[16–19] Regular surveillance is recommended throughout the pregnancy. Close observation for maternal hypertension and proteinuria, in addition to appropriate fetal growth surveillance with ultrasound, is advised in the second and third trimesters. Doppler assessments are widely used in Europe to assess for preeclampsia, placental insufficiency, and fetal growth restriction.[9]

Recent well-designed studies have been a welcome addition to previous recommended treatment. Aspirin is commonly used as a treatment for recurrent miscarriages, even those deemed idiopathic. Two randomized controlled trials have compared aspirin with placebo or supportive care in women with APS,[20,21] but no significant difference was found in the defined outcomes. A Cochrane review concluded that combined unfractionated heparin (UFH) and aspirin may reduce pregnancy loss by 54%, yet randomized controlled trials with adequate allocation concealment are needed to explore potential differences between UFH and low-molecular-weight heparin (LMWH).[22]

Two further well-designed studies comparing aspirin alone versus aspirin plus LMWH in women with APS found no differences in live birth rates and miscarriages.[23,24]

INFECTION

Infection seems to have a role in causing miscarriage in the mid-trimester rather than the first trimester.[25] A retrospective study of placental histology of more than 7000 spontaneous deliveries demonstrated histologic chorioamnionitis in 94% before

24 weeks' gestation compared with 40% between 25 and 28 weeks and 11% after 33 weeks.[26] Similar results were found in a case-control study, wherein chorioamnionitis was diagnosed in 77% of spontaneous MTLs compared with no infection found in the control group (induced labor for fetal anomaly).[27] However, the appearance of chorioamnionitis may well be secondary to a primary insult in an unknown number of cases previously described.

Microorganisms associated with preterm birth have been shown to play a key role in MTL. Chorioamnionitis involves organisms such as anaerobic streptococci, enterococci, coliforms, staphylococci, *Fusobacterium* spp, *Mycoplasma* spp, *Ureaplasma* spp, and group B β-hemolytic streptococci.[28] The most common pathway for an intrauterine infection is the ascent from the cervix and vagina.

Bacterial vaginosis is prevalent in up to 50% of pregnant women[29] and is considered a risk factor for PTD, PPROM, and MTL.[30] Bacterial vaginosis is an imbalance of vaginal flora caused by a reduction of the normal lactobacillary bacteria, and a heavy overgrowth of mixed anaerobic flora, including *Gardnerella vaginalis*, *Mycoplasma hominis*, and *Mobiluncus* species.

Classical diagnosis of BV[31] is known to be complex and time-consuming. A less strict inclusion system, the Nugent's classification, is now more widely used, because it includes an intermediate-flora classification characterized by abnormal genital-tract colonization that may represent a progression to full BV.[7] Ideally, an HVS should be performed in the first quarter of the menstrual cycle when levels are highest.[2]

Evidence shows that an intermediate-flora diagnosis has an association with adverse pregnancy outcome.[32] The influence of sexually transmitted diseases (STDs), with or without BV, on adverse pregnancy outcome has not been clearly defined.[33] Literature suggests that *Trichomonas vaginalis* is associated with BV and PPROM.[34] *Chlamydia trachomatis* in conjunction with BV has been found to increase the rate of PTL.[35]

TREATMENT

Treatment of intermediate abnormal vaginal flora and BV has been shown to reduce the occurrence of MTL.[36] Debate exists regarding the timing of optimal treatment of abnormal vaginal flora and BV. Results from 5 trials in the Cochrane review[4] are encouraging, showing a reduction in PTD when treated before 20 weeks. Commencing antibiotics early in the second trimester is highly recommended[37]; however, little research has been performed on the best possible route or dose.

Results of a large trial randomizing 624 women positive for BV and at high risk of PTD to either metronidazole and erythromycin or placebo showed that treatment with antibiotics reduced the rate of PTD.[38] The ORACLE II trial[39] compared the use of erythromycin and/or amoxicillin-clavulanate (co-amoxiclav) versus placebo in women in spontaneous preterm labor and intact membranes with no overt signs of clinical infection. The aim of the ORACLE Children Study II was to determine the long-term effects on children after exposure to antibiotics in this clinical situation. The authors advocate caution when using erythromycin in pregnancy due to an observed increase in the rate of cerebral palsy.[40] Used in isolation, metronidazole is less efficacious because of its narrow range of activity against BV organisms.

Clindamycin therapy for BV or intermediate vaginal flora, when initiated early in the second trimester, has been shown to significantly reduce MTL.[36,41,42] Two large randomized controlled trials used a course of either 300 mg of oral clindamycin[36] or 5 g of 2% intravaginal clindamycin pessaries.[41] Both studies emphasize the importance of early screening and treatment. The current preferred regimen is a 7-day course of 2% clindamycin cream vaginally (5 g of cream containing 100 mg of clindamycin phosphate).[43] Even though oral administration is straightforward, fewer systematic side effects may occur with the intravaginal route. Little evidence supports screening of the general obstetric population for BV and abnormal vaginal flora in the absence of a history of MTL/PTD.

UTERINE ANOMALY

Uterine anomalies can be grouped into congenital (disorders of the müllerian tract) or acquired (adhesions or leiomyomas). Although some uterine defects may have no impact on pregnancy outcome, others may contribute to miscarriage, intrauterine growth restriction, and PTL.[44,45]

CUAs are rare, and a lack of consistency exists regarding their clinical significance and optimal management. The true population prevalence is difficult to assess, because no universally accepted standardized classification system exists and diagnostic techniques tend to be invasive. As a result, prevalence rates in the literature can vary between 0.06% and 38.00%.

A recent literature review evaluating the presence of CUAs in high-risk women reported a prevalence of 13.3% among women with a history of miscarriage.[46] CUAs arise from the failure of the müllerian tract to complete bilateral duct elongation, fusion, canalization, or septal resorption of the müllerian ducts (**Table 2**).[47]

An abundance of studies have described CUA and miscarriage rates; however, few differentiate between early pregnancy loss and MTL. No specific study has researched unicornuate and bicornuate uterus in association with MTL.[5] A recent case-control study found that women with an arcuate uterus are not at any greater risk of MTL. Nonetheless, the study suggests a 3-fold increased risk of an MTL with a diagnosed septate or bicornuate uterus.[48] One hypothesis is that of an altered intrauterine pressure, not found in an arcuate uterus, that would contribute to subsequent myometrial and cervical dysfunction.[48] Further trials are required to explore the relationship between CUAs and MTL.

DIAGNOSIS

CUAs are typically diagnosed using ultrasound, hysterosalpingography, or under direct vision with hysteroscopy. Laparoscopy and magnetic resonance imaging can also be performed. Three-dimensional (3D) ultrasound has the advantage of being noninvasive and allows complete assessment of uterine morphology. Uterine dimensions can be measured, thus evaluating the likely success of any surgical intervention.[47] In several studies, 3D ultrasound has compared favorably to hysterosalpingography and laparoscopy for diagnosing CUAs.[49,50]

TREATMENT

Controversy surrounds the benefit of surgical uterine correction. Uncertainty exists about the efficacy of hysteroscopic surgical resection/metroplasty of the subseptate uterus. Although several uncontrolled small studies have claimed improvements in future pregnancies after resection,[51,52] no randomized controlled trials support these observations. An increased rate of obstetric complications has been described after hysteroscopic metroplasty, such as fetal malpresentation at term and an increased rate of delivery by caesarean section.[53]

Table 2 American Society of Reproductive Medicine (previously American Fertility Society) classification of anomalies of the müllerian duct		
Classification	Clinical Finding	Description
I	Segmental or complete agenesis or hypoplasia	Agenesis and hypoplasia may involve the vagina, cervix, fundus, tubes, or any combination Mayer-Rokitansky-Küster-Hauser syndrome is the most common example in this category
II	Unicornuate uterus with or without a rudimentary horn	When an associated horn is present, this class is subdivided into *communicating* (continuity with the main uterine cavity is evident) and *noncommunicating* (no continuity with the main uterine cavity) The noncommunicating type is further subdivided based on whether an endometrial cavity is present in the rudimentary horn
III	Didelphys uterus	Complete or partial duplication of the vagina, cervix, and uterus characterizes this anomaly
IV	Complete or partial bicornuate uterus	Complete bicornuate uterus is characterized by a uterine septum that extends from the fundus to the cervical os The partial bicornuate uterus demonstrates a septum, which is located at the fundus In both variants, the vagina and cervix each have a single chamber
V	Complete or partial septate uterus	A complete or partial midline septum is present within a single uterus
VI	Arcuate uterus	A small septate indentation is present at the fundus
VII	Diethylstilbestrol-related abnormalities	A T-shaped uterine cavity with or without dilated horns is evident

Adapted from The American Fertility Society classifications of adnexal adhesions, distal tubal occlusion, tubal occlusion secondary to tubal ligation, tubal pregnancies, müllerian anomalies and intrauterine adhesions. Fertil Steril 1988;49:944–55; with permission.

Outcomes are anticipated from The Randomised Uterine Septum Transection (TRUST) trial comparing hysteroscopic metroplasty and expectant management in the miscarriage population.[54]

CERVICAL WEAKNESS

True cervical weakness is an accepted cause for MTL and PTD, yet no universal consensus exists on the definition or appropriate diagnostic testing.[55,56] All other potential causes of MTL must be excluded, because consequential management is invasive and has associated risks. The inclusion criterion for the Cervical Incompetence Prevention Randomized Cerclage Trial (CIPRACT) was defined as "the initial, painless, progressive dilatation of the uterine cervix, where PTD seems inevitable without interference."[57] The diagnosis is made in the absence of other causes of PTD, such as uterine anomaly, fibroids, or infection, and only when singleton pregnancies are involved.[57] In the nonpregnant state, the passage, without resistance, of a size

9 Hegar dilator (Medline Industries, Inc., Mundelein, IL, USA) through the cervix, acts as a surrogate measure.[2] An accurate clinical event sequence is paramount to avoid the overuse of non–evidence-based, ineffective medicine and surgery.

MANAGEMENT
Ultrasound Assessment

Ultrasound assessment of cervical length has emerged as an effective prognosticator for PTD, especially in women with a previous history.[58] Transvaginal cervical length measurements are far superior and more reliable than digital cervical examination in assessing the length of the cervical canal, with an interobserver and intraobserver viability of less than 10%.[59]

The risk of adverse obstetric outcome is inversely related to the length of the cervix and the gestational age at detection of a short cervix. Cervical length of less than 25 mm has been found in most populations to have the best predictive accuracy for MTL/PTD, and may be the most reliable threshold to define a high-risk population.[60,61]

A large randomized study screened 47,000 low-risk women for cervical shortening at 23 weeks' gestation using transvaginal ultrasound.[62] Of these women, 470 had a cervical length measurement of 15 mm or less and were consequently randomized to either cerclage or expectant management. The incidence of PTD was similar in both groups, indicating that ultrasound-indicated cerclage is not beneficial in women who have an incidental finding of a short cervix, in the absence of a previous MTL/PTD.[63]

Conversely, women with a prior obstetric risk may benefit from an ultrasound finding of a short cervix. A meta-analysis of 4 randomized controlled trials showed that women with a previous MTL/PTD and a cervical length of less than 25 mm had a higher rate of pregnancies continuing into the third trimester after insertion of cerclage.[64] No studies have evaluated ultrasound-indicated cerclage performed in the presence of funneling. Cervical length measurement may also be useful in reassuring and monitoring women who have been treated with cerclage.

PROGESTERONE

Progesterone supplementation has been used for more than 50 years; however, scientific evidence supporting its efficacy is lacking. The hormone seems to have anti-inflammatory properties,[65] thus preventing cervical ripening.[66] Progesterone can be prescribed in the form of a vaginal pessary or gel, or as an intramuscular injection (17α-hydroxyprogesterone caproate). Extensive literature has described the use of progesterone in preventing PTD and recurrent miscarriages; however, none has focused on MTL in isolation. Two randomized controlled trials[67,68] and an individual patient data meta-analysis[69] have shown that the rate of PTD is reduced with the use of vaginal progesterone.

A recent comprehensive literature review of the use of vaginal progesterone and cervical cerclage in women with a sonographically short cervix found that these treatments have similar efficacy for preventing PTD. The authors propose that high-risk obstetric patients be treated with 17α-hydroxyprogesterone caproate from 16 weeks, followed by cervical length measurements beginning at 18 weeks. If the cervical length measurement is less than 25 mm, vaginal progesterone should be offered.[70]

No guidance exists on the use of progesterone in the prevention of MTL. Suggestions for proposed treatment regimens are extrapolated from studies detailing previous PTD or short cervical length. Research in the form of well-designed double-blind studies is required before progesterone supplementation can be evidence-based in the MTL cohort.

TRANSVAGINAL CERVICAL CERCLAGE

The goal of cerclage is to strengthen the internal cervical os to maintain a pregnancy. In the mid-20th century, Shirodkar[71] and McDonald[72] described the 2 classical techniques of transvaginal cervical cerclage (TVC). The difference in technique is that with a Shirodkar cerclage, the bladder is reflected to enable the suture to be placed as close to the internal cervical os as possible per vaginam. The choice of technique is usually at the discretion of the surgeon. Evidence shows no significant difference in PTD rates between the Shirodkar and McDonald techniques.[73]

RESEARCH EVIDENCE FOR TVC

Cerclage is a common prophylactic intervention for MTL and PTD, despite the lack of a well-defined population for whom evidence of a clear benefit exists. TVC is not without risks. The procedure is associated with an increased likelihood of medical intervention, hospital admission, puerperal pyrexia, induction of labor, and caesarean section.

The largest study to evaluate the efficacy of TVC included 1292 women at risk of PTD.[74] The authors concluded that women with a history of at least 3 previous MTLs were the only group to show a benefit from cerclage placement. The overall risk of PTD decreased from 32% to 15%. Similar results were found in a multicenter randomized controlled trial; however, the criterion for patient selection was the finding of a short cervix on routine transvaginal scanning at 22 weeks. Women with a cervix length of 15 mm or less were randomised to cerclage or expectant management. The PTD rate before 33 weeks was 22% in the cerclage group compared with 26% in the control group.[75]

The CIPRACT trial recruited 35 women with a history suggestive of cervical weakness and a cervical length measurement of less than 25 mm before 27 weeks' gestation. PTD before 34 weeks was 0% in women treated with cerclage compared with 44% in the control group. The authors concluded that therapeutic TVC with bedrest reduces PTD, but found no statistical difference in neonatal survival.[57] A further randomized controlled trial failed to show an improved perinatal outcome with TVC, suggesting that ultrasonographic dilatation of the internal os and shortening of the distal cervix is a consequence of pathophysiological processes such as inflammatory and infective stimuli.[76]

CERVICAL OCCLUSION

Total cervical occlusion involves closure of the external os using a continuous suture during the first trimester in addition to the primary TVC. The hypothesized action is that in conjunction with a TVC, which increases the resistance of a weakened cervix, a cervical mucus plug may prevent ascending infection, acting as a mechanical and immunologic barrier.[77] A recent multicenter, stratified, randomized controlled trial recruited 309 women to TVC with or without occlusion. The trial stopped early because of slow recruitment and an interim analysis that showed no benefit associated with occlusion in terms of gestational age at delivery and admission to the neonatal intensive care unit.[78]

"If cervical cerclage during gestation is indicated but the vaginal approach is impossible, why not accomplish constriction from above?"[79]

TRANSABDOMINAL CERCLAGE

Cases exist in which cervical cerclage has failed or is deemed inappropriate. Examples include the presence of a short or absent cervix after surgery, congenital deformity, and scarring as a consequence of obstetric trauma or previous cerclage. Benson and Durfee[79] first performed a transabdominal cerclage (TAC) in 1965 between 14 and 24 weeks' gestation. They first performed a midline incision, then opened the broad ligament, and, after mobilizing the uterine vessels, sought an avascular space through which to pass a 5-mm Mersilene tape.

A preconceptual interview is crucial for appropriate patient selection. Full disclosure and considerable explanation must be provided regarding the risks of failure, complications of insertion after previous surgery (eg, classical caesarean delivery; hourglass constriction of the cervix; damage to adjacent major blood vessels, bowel, or bladder), and the need for 2 major operations. This discussion should be followed by a second counseling appointment so the patient is fully informed and understands that a TAC is the last resort. Inclusion and exclusion criteria are described in **Table 3**. The procedure is outlined in **Box 1**.

RESEARCH EVIDENCE FOR TAC

Currently, no randomized studies have compared the effectiveness of TAC with expectant management or TVC.[63] A systematic review reported a lower delivery rate before 24 weeks' gestation in women with a TAC compared with those who had a repeat TVC.[80] These outcomes were reiterated in a further study in which TAC, rather than TVC, improved PTD rates.[81] Results should be viewed with caution, however, because assignment to either group was at the author's discretion, no prospective analysis was conducted, and several cases were excluded from the report.

No study has compared the insertion of TAC preconceptually or during pregnancy. In the nonpregnant state, the procedure is associated with fewer complications and the risk of bleeding is reduced. Some case reports have described a laparoscopic approach to TAC; however, currently no evidence suggests that it is superior.[63] In a recent multicenter cohort study, 66 preconceptual laparoscopic abdominal cerclages were performed in women with at least one pregnancy loss in the second or third

Table 3
Important preconceptual findings from history, full investigation protocol, and event sequence analysis

Inclusion Criteria	Exclusion Criteria
Elective vaginal cerclage for the treatment of cervical weakness failed, causing MTL	Multiple pregnancy
Completion of a full investigation protocol for MTL	Untreated coexisting cause of recurrent miscarriage
Cervical length measurement >20 mm on transvaginal ultrasound	Incomplete investigation protocol
Viable singleton pregnancy	Unwillingness to undergo randomization of treatment

Box 1
Transabdominal cerclage procedure

- Fetal viability confirmed through preprocedure scan (if performed during pregnancy)
- Preoperative thromboprophylaxis and intraoperative antibiotics administered
- Laparotomy performed between 9 and 13 weeks.
- Catheter placed in situ
- Vaginal pack placed to elevate uterus and improve access to cervico-isthmic region
- Patient placed in the Trendelenburg position
- Low transverse abdominal incision performed
- Peritoneum of the uterovesical fold incised transversely in the midline
- Uterine vessels and isthmus identified digitally
- Double-stranded 2-gauge nylon suture mounted onto a loose 40-mm round-bodied Mayo needle
- Isthmus grasped between thumb and forefinger to stabilize the uterus
- Suture inserted posteroanteriorly through the window between the substance of the cervix lateral to the canal but medial to the uterine vessels—the level of the uterine isthmus above the insertion of the uterosacral ligaments
- Needle remounted and procedure repeated posteroanteriorly on opposite side (**Fig. 3**)
- Knot tied anteriorly, covered by loose peritoneal fold
- Abdomen closed
- Inpatient stay 2 days
- Fetal viability scan performed before discharge
- TAC left in situ permanently

Adapted from Farquharson RG. Late pregnancy loss. In: Farquharson RG, Stephenson MD, editors. Early pregnancy. Cambridge (UK): Cambridge University Press; 2010. p. 277–86; with permission.

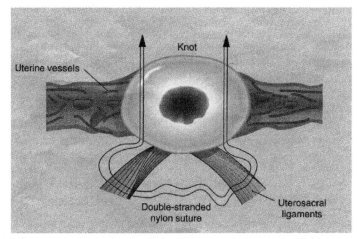

Fig. 3. Transabdominal cerclage technique. (*Adapted from* Farquharson RG. Late pregnancy loss. In: Farquharson RG, Stephenson MD, editors. Early pregnancy. Cambridge: Cambridge University Press; 2010. p. 277–86; with permission.)

trimester and/or a short or absent cervix. A total of 25 patients (71%) delivered after 34 weeks' gestation; however, 3 women experienced a further MTL. The perioperative complication rate was 4.5%. No mention was made of a thorough investigation protocol preceding the cerclage to exclude any other possible condition contributing to their poor obstetric history.[82] A case series of 40 TACs report a success rate of 90% (n = 36). The 4 cases with adverse outcomes had evidence of other pathologies contributing to the pregnancy loss (APS and chorioamnionitis).[83]

The presence of dual pathology, in conjunction with cervical weakness, is associated with a 56% risk of delivery before 34 weeks' gestation.[83] The authors emphasize the importance of comprehensive screening and counseling when considering a TAC, especially with a positive diagnosis of other MTL-associated conditions.

REFERENCES

1. Drakeley AJ, Quenby S, Farquharson RG. Mid-trimester loss–appraisal of a screening protocol. Hum Reprod 1998;13(7):1975–80.
2. Farquharson RG. Late pregnancy loss. In: Farquharson RG, Stephenson MD, editors. Early pregnancy. Cambridge (UK): Cambridge University Press; 2010. p. 277–86.
3. Wyatt PR, Owolabi T, Meier C, et al. Age-specific risk of fetal loss observed in a second trimester serum screening population. Am J Obstet Gynecol 2005;192: 240–6.
4. Flint S, Gibb DM. Recurrent second trimester miscarriage. Curr Opin Obstet Gynecol 1996;8:449–53.
5. Dukhovny S, Zutshi P, Abbott JF. Recurrent second trimester pregnancy loss: evaluation and management. Curr Opin Endocrinol Diabetes Obes 2009; 16(6):451–8.
6. McNamee K, Dawood F, Farquharson RG. Thrombophilia and early pregnancy loss. Best Pract Res Clin Obstet Gynaecol 2012;26(1):91–102.
7. McDonald HM, Brocklehurst P, Gordon A. Antibiotics for treating bacterial vaginosis in pregnancy. Cochrane Database Syst Rev 2007;(4):CD000262.
8. McNamee K, Dawood F, Farquharson RG. Evaluation of array comparative hybridization in recurrent miscarriage. Br J Hosp Med 2013;74(1):36–40.
9. Ruiz-Irastorza G, Crowther M, Branch W, et al. Antiphospholipid syndrome. Lancet 2010;376:1498–509.
10. Branch DW, Khamashta MA. Antiphospholipid syndrome: obstetric diagnosis, management and controversies. Obstet Gynecol 2003;101:1333–44.
11. Carp HJ. Thrombophilia and recurrent pregnancy loss. Obstet Gynecol Clin North Am 2006;33(3):429–42.
12. Pierangeli SS, Girardi G, Vega-Ostertag M, et al. Requirement of activation of complement C3 and C5 for antiphospholipid antibody-mediated thrombophilia. Arthritis Rheum 2005;52:2120–4.
13. Rai RS, Clifford K, Cohen H, et al. High prospective fetal loss rate in untreated pregnancies of women with recurrent miscarriages and antiphospholipid syndrome. Hum Reprod 1995;10(12):3301–4.
14. Branch DW, Scott JR, Kochenour NK, et al. Obstetric complications associated with the lupus anticoagulant. N Engl J Med 1985;313(21):1322–6.
15. Unander AM, Norberg R, Hahn L, et al. Anticardiolipin antibodies and complement in ninety-nine women with habitual abortion. Am J Obstet Gynecol 1987; 156(1):114–9.

16. Jauniaux E, Farquharson RG, Christianson OB, et al. Evidence-based guidelines for the investigation and medical treatment of recurrent miscarriage. Hum Reprod 2006;21:2216–22.
17. Miyakis S, Lockshin MD, Atsumi T, et al. International consensus statement on an update of the classification criteria and for definite antiphospholipid syndrome (APS). J Thromb Haemost 2006;4:295–306.
18. American College of Obstetricians and Gynecologists. ACOG practice bulletin. Management of recurrent pregnancy loss. Number 24, February 2001. (Replace Technical Bulletin Number 212. September 1995). American College of Obstetrics and Gynaecologists. Int J Gynaecol Obstet 2002;78:179–90.
19. Bates SM, Greer IA, Pabinger I, et al. American College of Chest Physicians. Venous thromboembolism, thrombophilia, antithrombotic therapy, and pregnancy: American College of Chest Physicians Evidence-Based Clinical Practice Guidelines (8th Edition). Chest 2008;133(Suppl 6):844S–86S.
20. Tulppala M, Marttunen M, Söderstrom-Anttila V, et al. Low-dose aspirin in prevention of miscarriage in women with unexplained or autoimmune related recurrent miscarriage: effect on prostacyclin and thromboxane A2 production. Hum Reprod 1997;12(7):1567–72.
21. Pattison NS, Chamley LW, Birdsall M, et al. Does aspirin have a role in improving pregnancy outcome for women with the antiphospholipid syndrome? A randomized controlled trial. Am J Obstet Gynecol 2000;183(4):1008–12.
22. Empson MB, Lassere M, Craig JC, et al. Prevention of recurrent miscarriage for women with antiphospholipid antibody or lupus anticoagulant. Cochrane Database Syst Rev 2005;(2):CD002859.
23. Farquharson RG, Quenby S, Greaves M. Antiphospholipid syndrome in pregnancy: a randomized controlled trial of treatment. Obstet Gynecol 2002;100:408–13.
24. Laskin CA, Spitzer KA, Clark CA, et al. Low molecular weight heparin and aspirin for recurrent pregnancy loss; results from the randomized controlled HepASA Trail. J Rheumatol 2009;36:279–87.
25. Oakeshott P, Hay P, Hay S, et al. Association between bacterial vaginosis or chlamydial infection and miscarriage before 16 weeks' gestation: prospective community based cohort study. BMJ 2002;325(7376):1334.
26. Russell P. Prevalence at delivery of histologic chorioamnionitis at different stages of gestation. Am J Diagn Gynec Obstet 1979;1:127.
27. Allanson B, Jennings B, Jacques A, et al. Infection and fetal loss in the mid-second trimester of pregnancy. Aust N Z J Obstet Gynaecol 2010;50(3):221–5.
28. Ugwumadu A. Chorioamnionitis and mid-trimester loss. Gynecol Obstet Invest 2010;70:281–5.
29. Nelson DB, Macones G. Bacterial vaginosis in pregnancy: current findings and future directions. Epidemiol Rev 2002;24:102–8.
30. Guerra B, Ghi T, Quarta S, et al. Pregnancy outcome after early detection of bacterial vaginosis. Eur J Obstet Gynecol Reprod Biol 2006;128:40–5.
31. Spiegel CA, Amsel R, Holmes KK. Diagnosis of bacterial vaginosis by direct gram stain of vaginal fluid. J Clin Microbiol 1983;18(1):170–7.
32. Hay PE, Lamont RF, Taylor-Robinson D, et al. Abnormal bacterial colonisation of the genital tract and subsequent preterm delivery and late miscarriage. BMJ 1994;308(6924):295–8.
33. Puwar M, Ughade S, Bhagat B, et al. Bacterial vaginosis in early pregnancy and adverse pregnancy outcome. J Obstet Gynaecol Res 2001;27(4):175–81.

34. Minkoff H, Grunebaum AN, Richard H, et al. Risk factors for prematurity and premature rupture of membranes. A prospective study of the vaginal flora in pregnancy. Am J Obstet Gynecol 1984;150:965–72.

35. Martius J, Krohn MA, Hiller SL, et al. Relationships of vaginal lactobacillus species cervical Chlamydia Trachomatis and bacterial vaginosis to preterm birth. Obstet Gynecol 1989;161:808–12.

36. Ugwumadu A, Manyonda I, Reid F, et al. Effect of early oral clindamycin on late miscarriage and preterm delivery in asymptomatic women with abnormal vaginal flora and bacterial vaginosis: a randomised controlled trial. Lancet 2003;361:983–8.

37. Adinkra PE, Lamont RF. Abnormal genital tract flora and pregnancy loss. In: Farquharson RG, editor. Miscarriage. Dinton (England): Mark Allen Publishing Ltd; 2002. p. 108–30.

38. Hauth JC, Goldenberg RL, Andrews WW, et al. Reduced incidence of preterm delivery with metronidazole and erythromycin in women with bacterial vaginosis. N Engl J Med 1995;333:1732–6.

39. Kenyon SL, Taylor DJ, Tarnow-Mordi W. Broad-spectrum antibiotics for spontaneous preterm labour: the ORACLE II randomised trial. The Lancet 2001; 357(9261):989–94.

40. Kenyon S, Pike K, Jones DR, et al. Childhood outcomes after prescription of antibiotics to pregnant women with spontaneous preterm labour: 7-year follow up of the ORACLE II trial. Lancet 2008;372(9646):1319–27.

41. Lamont RF, Duncan SL, Mandal D, et al. Intravaginal clindamycin to reduce preterm birth in women with abnormal genital tract flora. Obstet Gynecol 2003;101:516–22.

42. Lamont RF, Jones BM, Mandal D, et al. The efficacy of vaginal clindamycin for the treatment of abnormal genital tract flora in pregnancy. Infect Dis Obstet Gynecol 2003;11:181–9.

43. Workowski KA, Berman S. Sexually transmitted diseases treatment guidelines, 2010 Centers for Disease Control and Prevention (CDC). MMWR Recomm Rep 2010;59(RR-12):1.

44. Raga F, Bauset C, Remohi J, et al. Reproductive impact of congenital Müllerian anomalies. Hum Reprod 1997;12(10):2277–81.

45. Salim R, Regan L, Woelfer B, et al. A comparative study of the morphology of congenital uterine anomalies in women with and without a history of recurrent first trimester miscarriage. Hum Reprod 2003;18(1):162–6.

46. Chan YY, Jayaprakasan K, Zamora J, et al. The prevalence of congenital uterine anomalies in unselected and high risk populations: a systematic review. Hum Reprod Update 2011;17(6):761–71.

47. Devi Wold AS, Pham N, Arici A. Anatomic factors in recurrent pregnancy loss. Semin Reprod Med 2006;24(1):25–32.

48. Saravelos S, Cocksedge K, Li T. The pattern of pregnancy loss in women with congenital uterine anomalies and recurrent miscarriage. Reprod Biomed Online 2010;20(3):416–22.

49. Jurkovic D, Geipel A, Gruboeck K, et al. Three-dimensional ultrasound for the assessment of uterine anatomy and detection of congenital anomalies: a comparison with hysterosalpingography and two-dimensional sonography. Ultrasound Obstet Gynecol 1995;5(4):233–7.

50. Raga F, Bonilla-Musoles F, Blanes J, et al. Congenital Müllerian anomalies; diagnostic accuracy of three dimensional ultrasound. Fertil Steril 1996;65: 523–8.

51. Homer HA, Li TC, Cooke ID. The septate uterus: a review of management and reproductive outcome. Fertil Steril 2000;73(1):1–14.
52. Christiansen OB, Nybo Andersen AM, Bosch E, et al. Evidence-based investigations and treatments of recurrent pregnancy loss. Fertil Steril 2005;83(4):821–39.
53. Agostini A, De Guibert F, Salari K, et al. Adverse obstetric outcomes at term after hysteroscopic metroplasty. J Minim Invasive Gynecol 2009;16(4):454.
54. Kowalik CR, Mol BW, Veersema S, et al. Critical appraisal regarding the effect on reproductive outcome of hysteroscopic metroplasty in patients with recurrent miscarriage. Arch Gynecol Obstet 2010;282:465.
55. Berry CW, Brambatie B, Eskes T, et al. The Euro-Team Early Pregnancy (ETEP) protocol for recurrent miscarriage. Hum Reprod 1995;10(6):1516–20.
56. Ventolini G, Neiger R. Management of painless mid-trimester cervical dilation: prophylactic vs. emergency placement of cervical cerclage. J Obstet Gynaecol 2008;28(1):24–7.
57. Althuisius SM, Dekker GA, Hummel P, et al. Final results of the Cervical Incompetence Prevention Cerclage Trial (CIPRACT): therapeutic cerclage with bed rest versus bed rest alone. Am J Obstet Gynecol 2001;85:1106–12.
58. Owen J, Yost N, Berghella V, et al. Mid-trimester endo-vaginal sonography in women at risk for spontaneous preterm birth. JAMA 2001;286:1340–8.
59. Berghella V, Tolosa JE, Kuhlman KA, et al. Cervical Ultrasonography compared to manual examination as a predictor of preterm delivery. Am J Obstet Gynecol 1997;177:723–30.
60. Vidaeff AC, Ramin SM. Management strategies for the prevention of preterm birth: part II- update on cervical cerclage. Curr Opin Obstet Gynecol 2009;21:485–90.
61. Grimes-Dennis J, Berghella V. Cervical length and prediction of preterm delivery. Curr Opin Obstet Gynecol 2007;19:191–5.
62. To MS, Skentou C, Liao AW, et al. Cervical length and funneling at 23 weeks gestation in the prediction of spontaneous early preterm delivery. Ultrasound Obstet Gynecol 2001;8:200–3.
63. Abbott D, To M, Shennan A. Cervical cerclage: a review of current evidence. Aust N Z J Obstet Gynaecol 2012;52:220–3.
64. Berghella V, Odibo AO, To MS, et al. Cerclage for short cervix on ultrasonography: meta-analysis of trials using individual patient-level data. Obstet Gynecol 2005;106:181–9.
65. Elovitz MA, Gonzalez J. Medroxyprogesterone acetate modulates the immune response in the uterus, cervix and placenta in a mouse model of preterm birth. J Matern Fetal Neonatal Med 2008;21:223–30.
66. Xu H, Gonzalez JM, Ofori E, et al. Preventing cervical ripening: the primary mechanism by which progestional agents prevent preterm birth? Am J Obstet Gynecol 2008;198:314.e1–8.
67. Fonseca EB, Celik E, Parra M, et al. Progesterone and the risk of preterm birth among women with a short cervix. N Engl J Med 2007;357:462–9.
68. Hassan SS, Romero R, Vidyadhari D, et al. Vaginal progesterone reduces the rate of preterm birth in women with a sonographic short cervix: a multicenter, randomized, double-blind, placebo-controlled trial. Ultrasound Obstet Gynecol 2011;38:18–31.
69. Romero R, Nicolaides K, Conde-Agudelo A, et al. Vaginal progesterone in women with an asymptomatic sonographic short cervix in the midtrimester decreases preterm delivery and neonatal morbidity: a systematic review and metaanalysis of individual patient data. Am J Obstet Gynecol 2012;206:124.e1–19.

70. Conde-Agudelo A, Romero R, Nicolaides K, et al. Vaginal progesterone vs. cervical cerclage for the prevention of preterm birth in women with a sonographic short cervix, previous preterm birth, and singleton gestation: a systematic review and indirect comparison metaanalysis. Am J Obstet Gynecol 2013; 208(1):42.e1–18.

71. Shirodkar VN. A new method of operative treatment for habitual abortion in the second trimester. Antiseptic 1955;52:299–300.

72. McDonald IA. Suture of the cervix for inevitable miscarriage. J Obstet Gynaecol Br Emp 1957;64:346–50.

73. Odibo AO, Berghella V, To MS, et al. Shirodkar versus McDonald cerclage for the prevention of preterm birth in women with a short cervical length. Am J Perinatol 2007;24:55–60.

74. MRC/RCOG Working Party on Cervical Cerclage. Final report of the Medical Research Council/Royal College of Obstetricians and Gynaecologists multicentre randomized trial of cervical cerclage. Br J Obstet Gynaecol 1993;100: 516–23.

75. To MS, Alferivic Z, Heath VC, et al. Cervical cerclage for prevention of preterm delivery in women with short cervix: randomized controlled trial. Lancet 2004; 363:1849–53.

76. Rust OA, Atlas RO, Jones KJ, et al. A randomized trial of cerclage versus no cerclage among patients with ultrasonographically detected second trimester preterm dilatation of the internal os. Am J Obstet Gynecol 2000;183(4):830–5.

77. Hein M, Helmig RB, Schonheyder HD, et al. An in vitro study of antibacterial properties of the cervical mucus plug. Am J Obstet Gynecol 2001;185:586–92.

78. Brix N, Secher NJ, McCormack CD, et al. Randomised trial of cervical cerclage, with and without occlusion, for the prevention of preterm birth in women suspected of cervical insufficiency. Br J Obstet Gynaecol 2013;120(5):613–20.

79. Benson RC, Durfee RB. Transabdominal cervico-uterine cerclage during pregnancy for the treatment of cervical incompetence. Obstet Gynecol 1965;25: 145–55.

80. Zaveri V, Aghajafari F, Amankwah K, et al. Abdominal versus vaginal cerclage after a failed transvaginal cerclage: a systematic review. Am J Obstet Gynecol 2002;187:868–72.

81. Davis G, Berghella V, Talucci M, et al. Patients with a prior failed transvaginal cerclage: a comparison of obstetric outcomes with either transabdominal or transvaginal cerclage. Am J Obstet Gynecol 2000;183:836–9.

82. Burger NB, Einarsson JI, Brolmann HA, et al. Preconceptual laparoscopic abdominal cerclage: a multicentre cohort study. Am J Obstet Gynecol 2012; 207:273.e1–12.

83. Farquharson RG, Topping J, Quenby SM. Transabdominal cerclage: the significance of dual pathology and increased preterm delivery. BJOG 2005;112: 1424–6.

Endocrine Basis for Recurrent Pregnancy Loss

Raymond W. Ke, MD, HCLD

KEYWORDS

- Recurrent pregnancy loss • Luteal phase defect • Hyperprolactinemia
- Polycystic ovary syndrome • Thyroid disease • Thyroid antibodies

KEY POINTS

- Common endocrinopathies are a frequent contributor to both spontaneous and recurrent miscarriage.
- Although the diagnostic criteria for luteal phase defect is still controversial, treatment of patients with both recurrent pregnancy loss and luteal phase defect using progestogen in early pregnancy appears to be beneficial.
- With rising demand, an increase in thyroid gland function is critical in the maintenance of early pregnancy.
- Overt or subclinical hypothyroidism along with the presence of antithyroid antibodies is correlated with poor obstetric outcome.
- Women with polycystic ovary syndrome, the most common endocrinopathy of reproductive age women, have an increased risk of pregnancy loss.
- Management of hyperinsulinemia in polycystic ovary syndrome with normalization of weight or metformin appears to reduce the risk of pregnancy loss.

The human embryo enters the uterine cavity 4 days after ovulation. The process of implantation begins approximately 3 days later or typically between 19 and 23 days from the last menstrual cycle, a time period of high receptivity known as the *implantation window*.[1] It has been observed that the longer the ovulation-to-implantation interval, the higher the risk of early pregnancy loss.[2] Endocrine hormones play a critical role in the expression, modulation, and inhibition of various growth factors, cytokines, cell adhesions molecules, and decidual proteins. Estradiol and progesterone control the orderly growth and differentiation of the endometrium for implantation of the embryo. A receptive endometrium is characterized by growth and coiling of spinal arteries, secretory changes in the glands, and decidualization of the stromal compartment. Failure of the endometrium to respond to these hormonal signals can result in

The author has nothing to disclose.
Assisted Reproduction, Fertility Associates of Memphis, 80 Humphreys Center, Suite 307, Memphis, TN 38120, USA
E-mail address: rke@fertilitymemphis.com

Obstet Gynecol Clin N Am 41 (2014) 103–112
http://dx.doi.org/10.1016/j.ogc.2013.10.003
0889-8545/14/$ – see front matter © 2014 Elsevier Inc. All rights reserved.

defective placentation resulting in a risk of miscarriage. Recurrent pregnancy loss (RPL), defined as 2 or more consecutive pregnancy losses before the 20th week of pregnancy, is a frequent obstetric complication. One of the pathogenetic mechanisms underlying RPL includes a dysfunction of the endocrine system.

LUTEAL PHASE DEFECT

Crucial to the development of the endometrium is adequate glandular growth primarily mediated by abundant estradiol during the proliferative phase. At a threshold value, estradiol signals the pituitary to release a large amount of luteinizing hormone (LH) into circulation. This surge of circulating LH triggers oocyte maturation and release and the formation of the corpus luteum from the granulosa cells of the ruptured follicular bed. The luteal phase begins with the LH surge and ideally lasts 14 days in a nonpregnant menstrual cycle ending when hormone withdrawal from the involuting corpus luteum results in endometrial sloughing and the start of another menstrual cycle. Unique to the luteal phase is a sharp increase in progesterone production from the corpus luteum that, along with estradiol, peaks during the implantation window. Primarily through the action of progesterone, the endometrium undergoes stromal decidualization, and the glands switch to a secretory role in preparation for implantation.[3,4] A normal luteal phase is characterized by estradiol-mediated glandular growth in the preceding proliferative phase, adequate LH surge triggering ovulation, followed by robust progesterone production with an appropriate endometrial response.

Accordingly, the dysfunctional mechanisms resulting in luteal phase defect (LPD), also known as *luteal phase insufficiency*, may include poor follicular growth, oligo-ovulation, inadequate corpus luteum function, or altered endometrial response to secreted progesterone.[3] These mechanisms may arise from a wide spectrum of endocrinopathies and comorbidities such as hyperprolactinemia or stress (**Box 1**).[5] LPD has long been suspected with miscarriage and RPL.[6] However, quantifying the risk has been hampered by the difficulty in defining diagnostic criteria for LPD.[3,4] Although histologic dating of the endometrium after timed biopsy has been the historical gold standard for the diagnosis of LPD, the accuracy and reproducibility of this modality is highly suspect given significant intra- and interobserver variation in interpretation.[5,7] In a study of timed endometrial biopsies from 130 fertile women, Murray and colleagues[8] found that histologic endometrial dating had neither the accuracy nor the precision to diagnose LPD and thus did not help in the clinical management of these patients. A criterion of luteal phase length less than 11 days can be difficult to measure reliably and document consistently but could be useful as a screening evaluation for LPD. Luteal phase hormone levels, especially progesterone concentration, are more

---

Box 1
Identified causes of luteal phase defect

- Hyperprolactinemia
- Polycystic ovary syndrome
- Hypogonadotropic hypogonadism
- Poor ovarian reserve
- Stress
- Exercise
- Extreme weight loss

useful if performed serially over the course of the luteal phase to better identify peak levels. Regardless, hormone levels fluctuate significantly during the day and still may not reflect endometrial response to a given concentration.[9] Given the challenge of variable diagnostic criteria, the incidence of LPD in women with RPL is estimated between 12% and 28%.[10,11]

The lack of consensus in diagnostic criteria for LPD has made it difficult to arrive at management recommendations in RPL patients. Treatment options have varied widely and include luteal phase supplementation using progestogen or human chorionic gonadotropin (hCG), ovulation induction, or a combination of these. Medication types, doses, timing and routes of administration have remained contentious. Because a deficiency of progesterone action on the endometrium is arguably the critical feature of LPD, supplementing the luteal phase with pharmaceutical progestogens has remained the most common therapy. A Cochrane review of progestogen treatment in 15 studies found no statistical difference in miscarriage rates between progestogen or placebo groups.[12] However, when the analysis included only the 4 studies that identified women with 3 or more previous pregnancy losses, a statistically significant reduction of loss in the women randomly assigned to the progestogen-treated group (Peto odds ratio, 0.38; 95% confidence interval [CI], 0.20–0.70) was found (**Fig. 1**).

Hyperprolactinemia is a unique endocrinopathy that causes infertility and miscarriage through anovulation or, in more subtle forms, LPD. Elevated prolactin alters the hypothalamic-pituitary-ovarian axis leading to impaired folliculogenesis or a short luteal phase. Often, hyperprolactinemia is secondary to medication use or primary hypothyroidism. In these cases, correction of prolactin levels through management of the underlying cause should be attempted. Treatment of women with RPL and refractory hyperprolactinemia, with a dopamine agonist such as bromocriptine, significantly improved subsequent pregnancy outcome.[13]

THYROID DISEASE AND PREGNANCY LOSS

Normal pregnancy exerts a dramatic change in thyroid function and regulation. There is a marked demand for both thyroxine (T4) and triiodothyronine (T3) well greater than

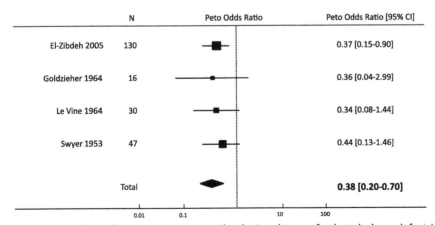

Fig. 1. Meta-analysis of progestogen versus placebo/no therapy for luteal phase defect in women with 3 or more previous miscarriages. (*Adapted from* Haas DM, Ramsey PS. Progestogen for preventing miscarriage. Cochrane Database Syst Rev 2008;(2):CD00351; with permission.)

that required in the nonpregnant state. Total T4/T3 concentrations increase sharply in early pregnancy and plateau early in the second trimester at concentrations 30% to 100% greater than prepregnancy values.[14] The increased demand for thyroid hormone in pregnancy predominantly arises from a 2- to 3-fold increase in circulating plasma thyroid binding globulin (TBG) binding to circulating T4/T3 reducing the pool of bioavailable hormone. TBG production is stimulated by estradiol from the corpus luteum and eventually the placenta. However, total T4/T3 is still less than would be expected by increased TBG binding resulting in an overall decline in free T4 during pregnancy. Greater demand for hormone production by the thyroid in pregnancy is also the result of deiodination of thyroxine by the placenta and the initial mild thyrotropic effects of human chorionic gonadotropin (**Fig. 2**). Therefore, if thyroid homeostasis is to be maintained in pregnancy, the gland must dramatically increase thyroid hormone production. The supply of dietary iodine, complicated further by the increase in renal iodide clearance, is crucial to allow increased production. Preexisting thyroid gland dysfunction may limit the ability of the gland to meet pregnancy demands.

Despite the known association between decreased fertility and hypothyroidism, the latter condition is not incompatible with conception. This is probably the main reason, until a few years ago, hypothyroidism had been considered—wrongly—to be rare during pregnancy. Abalovich and colleagues[15] observed that 34% of hypothyroid women became pregnant without T4 treatment. Of these, 11% suffered overt hypothyroidism, and 89% had subclinical hypothyroidism. Maternal thyroid-stimulating hormone (TSH) levels may decline in early pregnancy but otherwise should be maintained in the normal range through pregnancy. However, there is a debate regarding the normal upper limit of TSH. Whereas TSH values of 4.0 to 5.0 mIU/L were once considered normal, a consensus is emerging that a TSH value greater than 2.5 mIU/L is outside the normal range.[16]

If and when hypothyroid women become pregnant, they carry an increased risk for early and late obstetric complications (**Box 2**). A Dutch study of nearly 2500 pregnant women found that as TSH values increase—even in the usual normal range—there is an increased risk for fetal loss.[17] Endemic iodine deficiency is the most common cause

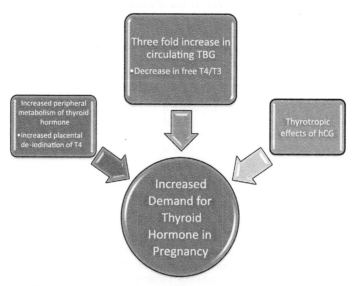

Fig. 2. Factors affecting demand for thyroid hormone in pregnancy.

Box 2
Adverse pregnancy outcomes of hypothyroidism

- Mother
  - Infertility
  - Miscarriage
  - Anemia
  - Preeclampsia
  - Abruptio placenta
- Baby
  - Fetal death
  - Preterm birth
  - Low birth weight
  - Impaired neurocognitive development

---

of hypothyroidism seen in pregnant women worldwide. Other causes include postsurgical, postradioiodine ablation and hypothyroidism secondary to pituitary disease such as lymphocytic hypophysitis. However, by far, the predominant etiology of hypothyroidism in iodine-replete populations is the spectrum of chronic autoimmune thyroid disease, often undiagnosed for years before presentation (**Box 3**). Among pregnant women, autoimmune thyroid disease has a prevalence of 5% to 20% depending on the population studied.[18] Women with antithyroid antibodies (ATA) during pregnancy have shown that, despite the expected decrease in antibody titers during gestation, thyroid function gradually deteriorated toward hypothyroidism in a significant fraction.[19] The most commonly targeted thyroid antigens are thyroperoxidase (TPO) and thyroglobulin (Tg), both integral to the production of T4 and T3. The reported prevalence of anti-TPO and anti-Tg antibodies in asymptomatic women is 14.6% and 13.8%, respectively.[20]

Stagnaro-Green and colleagues[21] first reported an association of ATA with RPL observing a doubling of the spontaneous miscarriage rate (17.0 vs 8.4%; $P = .001$)

Box 3
Autoimmune thyroid disease during pregnancy and the postpartum period

- Asymptomatic autoimmune disease
  - ATA positive; euthyroid
  - Subclinical hypothyroidism
- Primary hypothyroidism
  - Hashimoto's disease
  - TSH receptor–blocking antibody
- Grave's disease
  - Euthyroid
  - Hyperthyroid
  - Postpartum thyroiditis

in women with a TSH between 2.5 and 5.0 mIU/L who were ATA positive compared with an ATA-negative cohort. A pooled analysis of 21 studies (13 cohort and 8 case control) found an odds ratio (OR) of 2.55 (95% CI, 1.42–4.57; $P = .002$) for recurrent losses in women with ATA.[22] Similarly, a recent meta-analysis found a positive association of ATA with spontaneous pregnancy loss in both cohort (OR, 3.9; 95% CI, 2.48–6.12; $P<.001$) and case-control (OR, 1.8; 95% CI, 1.25–2.6; $P = .002$) studies.[23]

The precise pathogenetic link between ATA and pregnancy loss is unknown, and the association does not imply a causal relationship. Autoimmune thyroid disease may impair thyroid reserve to such an extent that the gland is unable to respond to the challenge of pregnancy. ATA may be associated with inappropriately low levels of thyroid hormones for the given gestational period, despite apparent biologic euthyroidism. Alternatively, autoimmune thyroid disease could act by delaying the occurrence of conception because of its known association with infertility. Similarly, women with autoimmune thyroid disease are generally older than healthy controls, and increased age is an independent risk factor for miscarriage. Finally, ATA may merely be a marker for a generalized immune imbalance, which may independently promote pregnancy loss.[18,24]

Regardless of the causal relationship, there is evidence that thyroid hormone replacement with levothyroxine in pregnant women with hypothyroidism (TSH >2.5 mIU/L), will improve pregnancy outcome.[15,25,26] Furthermore, a Cochrane study suggested a significant reduction in preterm birth and a trend toward reduced miscarriage when levothyroxine was used in euthyroid pregnant women with ATA.[27] Given that thyroid autoimmunity may be present for many years before the onset of hypothyroidism, it seems reasonable to test RPL patients for ATA (both anti-TPO and anti-Tg), preferably immediately before conception.[5] For those with positive antibodies and a TSH level greater than 2.5 mIU/L, levothyroxine therapy tailored to the TSH level is indicated.[26] Close monitoring, particularly in the first trimester, is important because of increasing thyroid demands with dosage often requiring titration upward during pregnancy.[28] There are no clear recommendations in ATA-positive pregnancies with a normal TSH (TSH <2.5 mIU/L), but common sense dictates that at the very least, close follow-up during pregnancy is warranted.

POLYCYSTIC OVARY SYNDROME

Although the exact prevalence is uncertain, women with polycystic ovarian syndrome (PCOS), have an increased frequency of pregnancy loss.[29] In the past, diagnostic criteria for this heterogeneous disorder have not been uniform, resulting in a wide range of reported prevalence of both miscarriage and RPL in PCOS patients.[30,31] In 2003, a consensus conference reached agreement on what has become known as the *Rotterdam Criteria* comprising oligo- or anovulation, hyperandrogenism, and ultrasonographic evidence of polycystic ovaries. PCOS is diagnosed with 2 of 3 defined criteria satisfied.[32] Notably absent from the consensus criteria is any reference to obesity or insulin sensitivity.

In the past, hypersecretion of LH and androgens have been linked to RPL.[33] Early observations have indicated an association between miscarriage and the elevated serum LH exhibited by many PCOS patients. However, there was no difference in subsequent pregnancy outcome in RPL women with high LH compared with those with normal LH.[33,34] Furthermore, there was no benefit seen in suppressing LH levels in PCOS patients with RPL.[35] Hyperandrogenism is considered by many investigators as the essential endocrinologic feature of PCOS. However, the association between excess androgens and the risk of RPL is also unclear. There was no observable difference in total testosterone values between women who miscarried and those with live birth.[34] Rai and colleagues[33] were unable to show that elevated testosterone levels in PCOS subjects were associated with an increased miscarriage rate. In contrast, Mulders and colleagues[36] and van Wely and colleagues[37] observed that lower total testosterone and a lower free androgen index in non-RPL women were more likely to have a successful pregnancy after ovulation induction.

A meta-analysis of 16 studies concluded that women with an increased body mass index have a significantly increased risk of miscarriage.[38] A body mass index greater than 30 kg/m^2 increases the chance of miscarriage by 20% and more than triples the risk of RPL development.[39] Many suffering from PCOS are obese and commonly found to exhibit metabolic disturbance involving insulin sensitivity. Hyperinsulinemia as a consequence of insulin resistance, an integral pathogenetic feature of PCOS, has emerged as a key factor behind the link between PCOS/obesity and the risk of RPL. Insulin resistance was found to be a significant independent risk factor for miscarriage in a study that investigated the fasting serum insulin concentrations before conception in 72 women with PCOS taking metformin.[40] Craig and colleagues[41] have observed increased insulin resistance in 27% of women with unexplained RPL and have recommended a determination of insulin metabolism as part of the evaluation of RPL. The connection between obesity and hyperinsulinemia with miscarriage may involve plasminogen activator inhibitor-1 (PAI-1), which inhibits plasmin formation during plasminogen activation and subsequent fibrinolysis. Elevated PAI-1 is reported to be an independent risk factor for pregnancy loss, potentially through a thrombophilic effect.[42–44]

In observational studies, the use of insulin-sensitizing agents such as metformin has reduced pregnancy loss in infertile, PCOS women with RPL when used before and throughout pregnancy.[29,45,46] In contrast, a randomized, placebo-controlled trial of metformin in infertile women did not find any benefit in preventing spontaneous pregnancy loss, but metformin was discontinued with the diagnosis of pregnancy.[47] It is still unclear if benefit could have been found if metformin was continued. Metformin has shown benefit in reducing the risk of miscarriage in women with a history of RPL and an abnormal glucose tolerance test result.[48] There is significant overlap among women with PCOS and type II diabetes mellitus. Uncontrolled type II diabetes is associated with an increased risk of pregnancy loss.[49] In a large, controlled, prospective study, early pregnancy loss was significantly correlated with elevated fasting glucose and glycosylated hemoglobin levels in the first trimester in insulin-dependent diabetics.[50] Metformin use during pregnancy does not appear to have any deleterious effects among exposed children studied during their first 18 months of life.[51] Of course, the alternative of losing weight in obese, anovulatory patients is also effective in improving insulin sensitivity and appears to improve fertility and pregnancy outcome.[52]

SUMMARY

Common endocrinopathies are a major contributor to both spontaneous and recurrent miscarriage. Although the diagnostic criteria for LPD are still controversial, treatment of patients with both RPL and LPD using progestogen in early pregnancy seems beneficial. Hyperprolactinemia, a unique cause of LPD, is easily evaluated and managed. An increase in thyroid gland function is critical in the maintenance of early pregnancy. Overt or subclinical hypothyroidism along with the presence of antithyroid antibodies is correlated with poor obstetric outcome. Thyroid hormone replacement therapy along with careful monitoring in the preconceptual and early pregnancy period is associated with improved outcome. Women with polycystic ovary syndrome, the most common endocrinopathy of reproductive age women, have an increased risk of pregnancy loss. The precise mechanism is unclear but likely involves hyperinsulinemia, a common feature of PCOS, possibly acting through the clotting factor PAI-1. Management of PCOS with normalization of weight or metformin seems to reduce the risk of pregnancy loss.

REFERENCES

1. Klentzeris LD. The role of the endometrium in implantation. Humanit Rep 1997; 12(Suppl 11):170–5.
2. Wilcox AJ, Baird DD, Weinberg CR. The time of implantation of the conceptus and loss of pregnancy. N Engl J Med 1999;340:1796–9.
3. Jones GS. The luteal phase defect. Fertil Steril 1976;27(4):351–6.
4. Noyes RW, Hertig AW, Rock J. Dating the endometrial biopsy. Fertil Steril 1950; 1:3–25.
5. Smith ML, Schust DJ. Endocrinology and recurrent pregnancy loss. Semin Reprod Med 2011;29:482–90.
6. Horta JL, Fernandez JG, de Leon BS, et al. Direct evidence of luteal insufficiency in women with habitual abortion. Obstet Gynecol 1977;49(6):705–8.
7. Saleh MI, Warren MA, Li TC, et al. A light microscopic morphometric study of the luminal epithelium of human endometrium during the peri-implantation period. Humanit Rep 1995;10:1828–32.
8. Murray MJ, Meyer WR, Zaino RJ, et al. A critical analysis of the accuracy, reproducibility, and clinical utility of histologic endometrial dating in fertile women. Fertil Steril 2004;81(5):1333–43.
9. Tulppala M, Björses UM, Stenman UH, et al. Luteal phase defect in habitual abortion: progesterone in saliva. Fertil Steril 1991;56(1):41–4.
10. Lessey BA, Fritz MA. Defective luteal function. In: Fraser JS, Jansen RP, Lobo RA, et al, editors. Estrogens and progestogens in clinical practice. Philadelphia: W.B. Saunders; 1998. p. 437–53.
11. Li TC, Spuijbroek MD, Tuckerman E, et al. Endocrinological and endometrial factors in recurrent miscarriage. BJOG 2000;107(12):1471–9.
12. Haas DM, Ramsey PS. Progestogen for preventing miscarriage. Cochrane Database Syst Rev 2008;(2):CD003511.
13. Hirahara F, Andoh N, Sawai K, et al. Hyperprolactinemic recurrent miscarriage and results of randomized bromocriptine treatment trials. Fertil Steril 1998;70: 246–52.
14. Glinoer D. The regulation of thyroid function in pregnancy: pathways of endocrine adaptation from physiology to pathology. Endocr Rev 1997;18:404–33.
15. Abalovich M, Gutierrez S, Alcaraz G, et al. Overt and subclinical hypothyroidism complicating pregnancy. Thyroid 2002;12:63–8.
16. Abalovich M, Amino N, Barbour LA, et al. Management of thyroid dysfunction during pregnancy and post partum: an Endocrine Society Clinical Practice guideline. J Clin Endocrinol Metab 2007;92(Suppl 8):S1–47.
17. Benhadi N, Wiersinga WM, Reitsma JB, et al. Higher maternal TSH levels in pregnancy are associated with increased risk for miscarriage, fetal or neonatal death. Eur J Endocrinol 2009;160(6):985–91.
18. Glinoer D. Thyroidal and immune adaptation to pregnancy: focus on maternal hypo- and hyperthyroidism. In: Lazarus J, Pirags V, Butz S, editors. The thyroid and reproduction. New York: Thieme; 2009. p. 36–58.

19. Glinoer D, Rihai M, Grün JP, et al. Risk of subclinical hypothyroidism in pregnant women with autoimmune thyroid disorders. J Clin Endocrinol Metab 1994;79: 197–202.
20. Hollowell JG, Staehling NW, Flanders WD, et al. Serum TSH, T(4), and thyroid antibodies in the United States population (1988 to 1994): national health and nutrition examination survey (NHANES III). J Clin Endocrinol Metab 2002; 87(2):489–99.
21. Stagnaro-Green A, Roman SH, Cobin RH, et al. Detection of at-risk pregnancy by means of highly sensitive assays for thyroid autoantibodies. J Am Med Assoc 1990;19:1422–5.
22. Chen L, Hu R. Thyroid autoimmunity and miscarriage: a meta-analysis. Clin Endocrinol 2011;74:513–9.
23. Thangaratinam S, Tan A, Knox E, et al. Association between thyroid autoantibodies and miscarriage and preterm birth: meta-analysis of evidence. BMJ 2011;342:d2616.
24. Kaprara A, Krassas GE. Thyroid autoimmunity and miscarriage. Hormones 2008;7:294–302.
25. Bussen S, Steck T, Dietl J. Increased prevalence of thyroid antibodies in euthyroid women with a history of recurrent in vitro fertilization failure. Humanit Rep 2000;15(3):545–8.
26. Negro R, Formosa G, Mangieri T, et al. Levothyroxine treatment in euthyroid pregnant women with autoimmune thyroid disease: effects on obstetrical complications. J Clin Endocrinol Metab 2006;91(7):2587–91.
27. Reid SM, Middleton P, Cossich MC, et al. Interventions for clinical and subclinical hypothyroidism pre-pregnancy and during pregnancy. Cochrane Database Syst Rev 2013;(5):CD00752.
28. Mandel SJ, Larsen PR, Seely EW, et al. Increased need for thyroxine during pregnancy in women with primary hypothyroidism. N Engl J Med 1990;323(2):91–6.
29. Glueck CJ, Wang P, Goldenberg N, et al. Pregnancy outcomes among women with polycystic ovary syndrome treated with metformin. Humanit Rep 2002; 17(11):2858–64.
30. Rai R, Clifford K, Regan L. The modern preventative treatment of recurrent miscarriage. Br J Obstet Gynaecol 1996;103:106–10.
31. Ford HB, Schust DJ. Recurrent pregnancy loss: etiology, diagnosis and therapy. Rev Obstet Gynecol 2009;2:76–83.
32. Rotterdam ESHRE/ASRM-Sponsored PCOS Consensus Workshop Group. Revised 2003 consensu diagnostic criteria and long-term health risks related to polycysic ovary syndrome. Fertil Steril 2004;81(1):19–25.
33. Rai R, Backos M, Rushworth F, et al. Polycystic ovaries and recurrent miscarriage - a reappraisal. Humanit Rep 2000;15:612–5.
34. Nardo LG, Rai R, Backos M, et al. High serum luteinizing hormone and testosterone concentrations do not predict pregnancy outcome in women with recurrent miscarriage. Fertil Steril 2002;77:348–52.
35. Clifford K, Rai R, Watson H, et al. Does suppressing luteinising hormone secretion reduce the miscarriage rate? Results of a randomised controlled trial. BMJ 1996;312:1508–11.
36. Mulders AG, Eijkemans MJ, Imani B, et al. Prediction chances for success or complications in gonadotrophin ovulation induction in normogonadotropic anovulatory infertility. Reprod BioMed Online 2003;7:170–8.
37. van Wely M, Bayram N, van der Veen F, et al. Predicting ongoing pregnancy following ovulation induction with recombinant FSH in women with polycystic ovary syndrome. Humanit Rep 2005;20:1827–32.

38. Metwally M, Ong KJ, Ledger WL, et al. Does high body mass index increase the risk of miscarriage after spontaneous and assisted conception? A meta-analysis of the evidence. Fertil Steril 2008;90(3):714–26.
39. Lashen H, Fear K, Sturdee DW. Obesity is associated with increased risk of first-trimester and recurrent miscarriage: matched case-control study. Humanit Rep 2004;19(7):205–10.
40. Maryam K, Bouzari Z, Basirat Z, et al. The comparison of insulin resistance frequency in patients with recurrent early pregnancy loss to normal individuals. BMC Res Notes 2012;5:133.
41. Craig LB, Ke RW, Kutteh WH. Increased prevalence of insulin resistance in women with a history of recurrent pregnancy loss. Fertil Steril 2002;78:487–90.
42. Atiomo WU, Bates SA, Condon JE, et al. The plasminogen activator inhibitor system in women with polycystic ovary syndrome. Fertil Steril 1998;69(2):236–41.
43. Glueck CJ, Wang P, Bornovali S, et al. Polycystic ovary syndrome, the G1691A factor V Leiden mutation, and plasminogen activator inhibitor activity: assocaition with recurrent pregancy loss. Metabolism 2003;52(12):1627–32.
44. Sun L, Lv H, Wei W, et al. Angiotensin-converting enzyme D/I and plasminogen activator inhibitor-1 4G/5G gene polymorphisms are associated with increased risk of spontaneous abortions in polycystic ovarian syndrome. J Endocrinol Invest 2010;33:77–82.
45. Glueck CJ, Phillips H, Cameron D, et al. Continuing metformin throughout pregnancy in women with polycystic ovary syndrome appears to safely reduce first-trimester spontaneous abortion: a pilot study. Fertil Steril 2001;75(1):46–52.
46. Jakubowicz DJ, Iuorno MJ, Jakubowicz S, et al. Effects of metformin on early pregnancy loss in polycystic ovary syndrome. J Clin Endocrinol Metab 2002;87(2):524–9.
47. Legro RS, Barnhart HX, Schlaff WD, et al. Cooperative multicenter reproductive medicine network. Clomiphene, metformin or both for infertility in the polycystic ovary syndrome. N Engl J Med 2007;356(6):551–66.
48. Zolghadri J, Tavana Z, Kazerooni T, et al. Relationship between abnormal glucose tolerance test and history of previous recurrent miscarriages, and beneficial effects of metformin in these patients: a prospective clinical study. Fertil Steril 2008;90(3):727–30.
49. Jovanovic L, Knopp H, Kim H, et al. Elevated pregnancy losses at high and low extremes of maternal glucose in early normal and diabetic pregnancies: evidence for a protective adaptation in diabetes. Diabetes Care 2005;28:1113–7.
50. Mills JL, Simpson JL, Driscoll SG, et al. Incidence of spontaneous abortion among normal women and insulin-dependent diabetic women whose pregnancies were identified within 21 days of conception. N Engl J Med 1988;319(25):1617–23.
51. Glueck CJ, Goldenberg N, Pranikoff J, et al. Height, weight and motor-social development during the first 18 months of life in 126 infants born to 109 mother with polycystic ovary syndrome who conceived on and continued metformin through pregnancy. Humanit Rep 2004;19(6):1323–30.
52. Clark AM, Ledger W, Galletly C, et al. Weight loss results in significant improvement in pregnancy and ovulation rates in anovulatory obese women. Humanit Rep 1995;10(10):2705–10.

Antiphospholipid Antibody Syndrome

William H. Kutteh, MD, PhD, HCLD[a,b,*], Candace D. Hinote, MD[c]

KEYWORDS

- Antiphospholipid syndrome • Antiphospholipid antibodies
- Recurrent pregnancy loss • Fetal demise • Unfractionated heparin
- Complications of pregnancy

KEY POINTS

- Antiphospholipid antibodies (aPLs) are acquired antibodies directed against negatively charged phospholipids, a group of inner and outer cell membrane antigens found in mammals.
- Obstetric antiphospholipid antibody syndrome (APS) is diagnosed in the presence of certain clinical features in conjunction with positive laboratory findings.
- Although obstetric APS was originally reported in association with slow progressive thrombosis and infarction in the placenta, it is most often associated with a poor obstetric outcome.
- Several pathophysiologic mechanisms of action of aPLs have been described.
- The most common histopathologic finding in early pregnancy loss has been defective endovascular decidual trophoblastic invasion.
- Treatment with heparin and aspirin is emerging as the therapy of choice, with approximately 75% of treated women with RPL and aPL having a successful delivery, compared with less than 30% without treatment.

INTRODUCTION

Antiphospholipid antibodies (aPLs) are acquired antibodies (immunoglobulin [Ig] G, IgM, and/or IgA isotypes) that react against negatively charged phospholipids. They were originally associated with a slow progressive thrombosis and infarction in the placenta[1] and thus have been classified as thrombophilic factors. aPLs should additionally be classified as autoimmune factors when considering implantation and

The authors have nothing to disclose.
^a Department of Obstetrics and Gynecology, Vanderbilt University Medical Center, Nashville, TN, USA; ^b Fertility Associates of Memphis, PLLC, 80 Humphreys Center, Suite 307, Memphis, TN 38120, USA; ^c MidSouth OB GYN, 6215 Humphreys Boulevard, Suite 100, Memphis, TN 38120, USA
* Corresponding author. Fertility Associates of Memphis, PLLC, 80 Humphreys Center, Suite 307, Memphis, TN 38120.
E-mail address: wkutteh@fertilitymem.com

Obstet Gynecol Clin N Am 41 (2014) 113–132
http://dx.doi.org/10.1016/j.ogc.2013.10.004
0889-8545/14/$ – see front matter © 2014 Elsevier Inc. All rights reserved.

pregnancy because of the complex nature of the interaction of aPLs with target tissues. They have been shown to inhibit the release of human chorionic gonadotropin from human placental explants; to block in vitro trophoblast migration, invasion, and multinucleated cell formation; inhibit trophoblast cell adhesion molecules; and to activate complement on the trophoblast surface, inducing an inflammatory response.[2–5]

Antiphospholipid syndrome (APS) is an autoimmune condition characterized by the production of aPL combined with certain clinical features. The presence of aPL (including anticardiolipin [aCL] and lupus anticoagulant [LAC]) during pregnancy is a major risk factor for adverse pregnancy outcome.[6] In large meta-analyses of studies of couples with recurrent pregnancy loss (RPL), the incidence of APS was between 15% and 20% compared with about 5% in nonpregnant women without a history of obstetric complications.[7,8] It is not yet understood how aPLs arise in patients with APS. Genetic factors and infection may play a role. Family studies suggest a genetic disposition to APS, either when it presents as a primary condition or when it is seen in the context of systemic lupus erythematosus (SLE). This genetic disposition is accounted for, at least in part, by the major histocompatibility complex. The antibodies generated in patients with APS seem to recognize epitopes on phospholipid-binding proteins, unlike the antibodies that arise following infections such as syphilis and Lyme disease, which recognize phospholipids directly.[9]

DIAGNOSIS OF APS

APS is a syndrome that is defined based on both clinical and laboratory criteria. The diagnosis can be based on the presence of the clinical manifestation together with the laboratory detection of abnormal antibodies (**Box 1**). APS is designated as primary in patients without clinical or laboratory evidence of an underlying condition or disease, and secondary when it is associated with other diseases or conditions.[10] SLE is the disorder in which APS is most commonly associated but it may be associated with other conditions.[11,12] **Box 2** lists the conditions associated with secondary APS that may be relevant to obstetricians.

Widespread interest in APS among all areas of medicine led to the First International Symposium on Antiphospholipid Antibodies in 1984. The purpose of this group was to bring together the international research and clinical communities with the goal of clinical and scientific sharing and standardization of APS. Meetings have been held periodically with research and clinical data reviewed and discussed at preconference meetings and committees. An article was published with the latest suggested criteria for the diagnosis of APS with the current version referred to as the Sydney criteria.[13] These criteria should be useful for research investigations because the criteria result in specific diagnoses; however, in the clinical setting, these criteria are not very sensitive. These committee recommendations have been widely published, but the committee is not sanctioned or supported by any governing body such as the American College of Obstetricians and Gynecologists. The committee is primarily composed of rheumatologists, hematologists, and internists, with minor representation from obstetricians.

Clinical Criteria

The clinical manifestations of primary and secondary APS are diverse and may involve most organ systems.[10,14] Based on currently available evidence, vaso-occlusive disease is the pathologic basis for many of the complications of primary and secondary APS. Therefore, preconception counseling of the patient with APS regarding the risks

Box 1
Clinical and laboratory criteria established for the research of definite antiphospholipid syndrome: the Sydney criteria

Note: At least 1 clinical and 1 laboratory criterion must be present for definite APS.

Clinical criteria

1. Vascular thrombosis

  One or more clinical episodes of an arterial, venous, or small vessel thrombosis, confirmed by imaging or Doppler studies or histopathology, without significant evidence of inflammation in the vessel wall.

2. Obstetric morbidity

  a. One or more unexplained demise of a morphologically normal fetus at or beyond 10 weeks of gestation, or

  b. One or more premature births of a morphologically normal neonate at or before 34 weeks of gestation, caused by severe preeclampsia or severe placental insufficiency, or

  c. At least 3 unexplained, consecutive miscarriages of less than 10 weeks of gestation. Known factors associated with recurrent miscarriage, including parental genetic, anatomic, and endocrinologic factors, should be ruled out.

Laboratory criteria

1. aCL IgG and/or IgM in blood, present in medium or high titers (greater than 40 GPL or MPL or greater than the 99th percentile) on 2 or more occasions at least 12 weeks apart, measured by a standardized ELISA.

2. Anti-β2GP1 antibody of IgG and/or IgM isotype in blood (greater than the 99th percentile) on 2 or more occasions at least 12 weeks apart, measured by a standardized ELISA.

3. Lupus anticoagulant present in plasma, on 2 or more occasions at least 12 weeks apart, detected according to the guidelines of the International Society on Thrombosis and Hemostasis, which include the following steps:

  a. Prolonged phospholipid-dependent coagulation using a screening test such as the aPTT, kaolin clotting time, dilute Russell viper venom time, and dilute prothrombin time

  b. Failure to correct the prolonged coagulation time on the screening test by mixing with normal plasma

  c. Shortening or correction of the prolonged coagulation time on the screening test by the addition of excess phospholipid or platelets

  d. Exclusion of other coagulopathies (eg, factor VIII inhibitor) or heparin

Adapted from Werner E, Lockwood C. Thrombophilias and Stillbirth. Clin Obstet Gynecol 2010;53:617–27; with permission.

for serious medical problems is essential. In women referred to reproductive endocrinologists with APS and histories of early loss, the prevalence of prior thromboembolic events is low. However, these patients are still at risk for thromboembolic events. Estrogen-containing oral contraceptive pills should be avoided in women with repeated positive aPL.[15] Furthermore, women should be counseled that a single low-dose aspirin (81 mg) per day may decrease this future risk for thromboembolic event, as suggested by Silver and colleagues.[16] Thus, it is important for clinicians to be cognizant of the red flags, which are indications to perform diagnostic testing for the LAC and aCL antibodies (**Box 3**).

Box 2
Classification of the APS relevant to obstetricians

I. Primary APS

    Obstetric antiphospholipid syndrome

II. Secondary APS

   A. Autoimmune disease

       SLE

       Rheumatoid arthritis

       Sjögren syndrome

       Systemic sclerosis

       Diabetes mellitus

       Crohn disease

       Autoimmune thyroid disease

   B. Malignancies

       Carcinoma of ovary and cervix

       Lymphoma

       Leukemia

   C. Drug-induced conditions

       Oral contraceptives

   D. Infectious diseases

       Syphilis

       Human immunodeficiency virus infection

Box 3
Indications to identify LAC and aPL in obstetric patients

RPL

Unexplained second-trimester or third-trimester loss

Fetal demise

Early-onset, severe preeclampsia

Pregnancy-related thrombosis (venous or arterial)

Severe IUGR

Autoimmune or connective tissue disease

False-positive serologic test for syphilis (Venereal Disease Research Laboratory or rapid plasma reagin)

Prolonged coagulation studies

Positive autoantibody tests

Laboratory Criteria

Lupus anticoagulant is an immunoglobulin (usually IgG, IgM, or both) that interferes with one or more of the phospholipid-dependent tests of in vitro coagulation.[17] The name is a misnomer in 2 ways. Although it is called an anticoagulant, patients with LAC more frequently have a hypercoagulable state. Second, LAC is frequently found in patients without SLE. The most common tests that have been used to identify the LAC include the activated partial thromboplastin time (aPTT), the kaolin clot time (KCT), the dilute Russell viper venom time (dRVVT), and the plasma clot time (PCT).

The advantages, disadvantages, and sensitivity of the screening procedures used for LAC are listed in **Table 1**. aPTT reagents vary widely in their sensitivity to LAC because of variations in the phospholipid present in the reagent. It is not a reliable test to use in pregnancy because coagulation proteins, which increase during pregnancy (fibrinogen, factor VIII, von Willebrand factor, factor VII, and factor X), may mask the LAC. The KCT is reliable and sensitive but cannot be used as a confirming test. The dRVVT is a sensitive test and, because the snake venom activates factor X, this test is less affected by pregnancy.[18]

Regardless of which test is used, there are 3 steps that are necessary to identify an LAC. Once a prolonged in vitro coagulation test has been identified, it is necessary to document the presence of an inhibitor. Most commonly, mixing studies are done with pooled normal platelet-poor plasma and patient plasma in a 1:1 ratio. In general, a marked prolonged aPTT corrects to nearly the value of normal plasma (within 5 seconds) if the abnormal coagulation test was caused by a factor deficiency. To confirm that the persistently prolonged aPTT is caused by the LAC, a confirmatory test, such as the platelet neutralization test, must be performed. Frozen, thawed

Table 1
Screening tests for lupus anticoagulants

Test	Variables Affected by Pregnancy	Advantages	Disadvantages	Sensitivity
aPTT	Increased factor VIII may mask	Readily available, easily automated, can be used in PL confirmatory step	Reagents vary widely in sensitivity to LAC	Least
KCT	Not significantly affected by pregnancy	Very sensitive to LAC if patient is on oral anticoagulants	Very sensitive to residual platelets; not readily automated; cannot use in PL confirmation step	Most
dRVVT	Not significantly affected by pregnancy	Easy to perform; readily available	Manual techniques, affected by heparin or oral contraceptives	Good
PCT	Increased factor VII may blunt LAC effect	Requires no reagents or equipment	Must be performed on freshly drawn blood; manual technique	Good

Adapted from Branch DW, Silver RM, Blackwell JL, et al. Outcome of treated pregnancies in women with antiphospholipid syndrome: an update of the Utah experience. Obstet Gynecol 1992;80:614–20; with permission.

platelets contain and release excess phospholipid, which is added to the patient plasma. The LAC is absorbed to the phospholipid and the in vitro coagulation test returns toward normal.[17]

aPLs are acquired antibodies (IgG, IgM, and/or IgA) that belong to the large family of antibodies that react against negatively charged phospholipids, including cardiolipin (diphosphatidyl glycerol), phosphatidylserine, phosphatidylinositol, and phosphatidylglycerol. In 1983, Harris introduced a solid phase immunoassay for cardiolipin.[19] Two years later, he developed an enzyme-linked immunosorbent assay (ELISA) for cardiolipin, which remains the gold standard. In this immunoassay, cardiolipin, phosphatidylserine, and other phospholipids are used as coating antigens on microtiter plates. There have been 3 international workshops to standardize reporting. Standards for cardiolipin IgG, IgM, and IgA are commercially available through the Antiphospholipid Laboratory, Inc. These standard sera have been assigned numerical values based on their ability to bind 1 μg of cardiolipin and the units are reported as IgG phospholipid units (GPL). Based on the original studies and recommendations of Harris,[7] positive values are considered greater than or equal to 20 GPL, greater than or equal to 20 IgM phospholipid units (MPL), and greater than or equal to 30 IgA phospholipid units (APL), respectively. It has been recommended that values be reported in a semiquantitated fashion such as negative, borderline, positive, and high positive. Positive tests should ideally be confirmed in 6 to 8 weeks. In general, aPLs decline during pregnancy, perhaps because of increase maternal blood volume and dilution. However, aPLs may increase in as many as 20% of women during pregnancy.

A major target molecule for aPL binding seems to be beta-2 glycoprotein-1 (β2GP1) present on the surface of trophoblastic cell membranes.[20,21] β2GP1 is a cationic plasma protein that is bound to phosphatidylserine, which is exposed on the surface of trophoblastic cell membranes undergoing syncytial formation. Although the physiologic role of β2GP1 is unclear, the molecule seems to inhibit thrombosis by reducing the conversion of prothrombin to thrombin on platelets and inhibiting the activation of the intrinsic coagulation cascade.[22] β2GP1 was added to the criteria for the definitive diagnosis of APS in the Sydney criteria[13]; it is thought to be a more specific indicator of APS but several studies indicate that it is less sensitive than aCL or aPL for the diagnosis of APS.

OBSTETRIC COMPLICATIONS OF APS

Determining the diagnosis of APS in an individual patient requires both laboratory and clinical criteria to be met. The most recent compelling data for a link between aPLs and pregnancy complications come from studies in women with recurrent miscarriage,[23,24] although data associated with fetal loss, severe preeclampsia before 34 weeks' gestation, and severe placental insufficiency are also increasing.[25]

Recurrent Pregnancy Loss

RPL has been defined as 2 or 3 or more consecutive losses before the 20th week of gestation with the same partner, and affects up to 2% to 4% of pregnancies.[26,27] However, requiring 3 failed pregnancies before initiating a work-up may offer little additional clinical insight compared with testing after the second loss.[27,28] The risk of miscarriage in subsequent pregnancies is 30% after 2 losses and 45% after 3 losses in patients without a history of live birth, therefore testing after 2 consecutive losses may spare the affected couple the difficulty of dealing with an additional failed pregnancy, and may minimize excessive and unproductive evaluation. The American

Society of Reproductive Medicine recently defined RPL as 2 or more failed clinical pregnancies as documented by ultrasonography or histopathologic documentation of products of conception to address this point, and recommended a thorough evaluation of RPL after two or more clinical losses.[27] It has been observed that circulating aPLs is the main risk factor in 7% to 25% of early RPL (loss in the first trimester), whereas prevalence studies show that between 1% and 5% of patients have LAC.[29,30] The failure rate of pregnancies when APS is strictly defined as aPL levels of greater than the 99% of a normal population is estimated to be up to 90% (52% of early miscarriages and 38% of late fetal loss). Patients positive for aPL with a first unexplained pregnancy loss before the 10th week of gestation are likely to experience a high-risk second pregnancy.[31] Although all 3 of the laboratory criteria for diagnosis of APS (the presence of LAC, increased levels of aCL antibodies, and increased levels of β2GP1[13]) have been linked with RPL, the risk varies with the different types of antibodies. For example, the presence of aCL antibodies is associated with an odds ratio (OR) of 22.6 (95% confidence interval, 5.7–8.9) for subsequent pregnancy loss, and the presence of β2GP1 antibodies increases the chance of recurrent miscarriage from 6.8% to 22.2% compared with women with LAC or aCL.[32]

As the literature confirmed the strong association between aPL antibodies and RPL, and as a better understanding of the pathogenic concepts of APS and fetal loss have been reported,[33] the obvious results have been attempts to use this knowledge to develop therapies for this common complication of pregnancy. Although low-dose aspirin plus heparin has been shown to reduce pregnancy loss rates in patients with RPL, the optimal dose and regimen continue to be investigated as recent reports indicate.[34,35] Based on these recent studies, it is becoming clear that, although live birth rates are improving with therapy, older studies suggest that these patients are still at risk for late pregnancy complications including stillbirth, early-onset preeclampsia, and intrauterine growth restriction (IUGR).[36,37]

Fetal loss

Late fetal loss (after 10 weeks of pregnancy) associated with aPL antibodies is one of the diagnostic criteria for APS,[13] with aCL antibodies and β2GP1 antibodies, but not LAC, being strongly associated with intrauterine fetal death.[32,38,39] Late fetal loss is also more common as the number of aPL antibody tests become positive. In a recent report from Italy involving 97 pregnancies in 79 patients with APS and without hereditary thrombophilia, triple positivity conferred a risk of late fetal loss of 52.6% compared with a loss rate of 2.2% when only 2 tests were positive.[40] This observation again highlights the potential importance of other aPLs as a part of the diagnostic evaluation for RPL.

Information regarding the association between APS and stillbirth (defined as an intrauterine fetal death at a minimum gestational age of 20 weeks) is less well defined, and only a few articles have specifically commented on APS and stillbirth. Therapy for patients with a prior stillbirth and APS with low-dose aspirin and heparin is commonly used but not supported by large-scale randomized controlled trials.[41]

Severe preeclampsia before 34 weeks

Another clinical criterion that defines APS is a preterm birth resulting from severe preeclampsia at or before 34 weeks of gestation, and different methodologies have been used to document this association. When using the International Classification of Diseases, Ninth Revision, Clinical Modification (ICD-9-CM) code for the aPL syndrome (795.79) in a hospital discharge dataset to investigate the presence of APS in a large (141,286) group of women who delivered in Florida in 2001, APS had an increased adjusted OR for preeclampsia and eclampsia at any gestational age of 2.93 (95% confidence interval, 1.51–5.69).[42] A systematic review and meta-analysis of 64 full-text studies that yielded 12 studies for analysis concluded in 2010 that the pooled OR for the association of aCL antibodies alone with preeclampsia was 2.86 (95% confidence interval, 1.37–5.98), and for severe preeclampsia (95% confidence interval, 2.66–46.75) was 11.15.[43]

This study again reported preeclampsia at all gestational ages and made no recommendations regarding screening for aCL antibodies in the presence of preeclampsia. A recent review in 2011 of APS and preeclampsia reported a rate of 20% of patients with severe preeclampsia before 34 weeks having at least 1 aPL test positive compared with 6% in late-onset (after 34 weeks' gestation) preeclampsia.[44] These results compare favorably with controlled cohort studies reviewed in that article, and the investigators conclude that, in the patient with severe preeclampsia at less than 34 weeks' gestation, testing should be done for LAC, aCL antibodies, and β2GP1 antibodies. Reinforcing the concern expressed earlier, Branch and colleagues[45] observed that 50% of women with APS develop preeclampsia despite treatment of early-onset pregnancy complications. In the past, many of these patients were treated with steroids, which have been shown to increase the frequency of gestational hypertension, gestational diabetes, and preterm delivery.[46,47] More recent studies that used heparin for the treatment of women with APS have not reported the same high frequency of late pregnancy complications.[34,35,48,49]

Severe Placental Insufficiency

Severe placental insufficiency, another clinical criterion of the APS, is the least well-defined criterion, and usually includes IUGR and abruptio placenta at or before 34 weeks' gestation. Using the 2001 Florida dataset described earlier, placental insufficiency (as defined by ICD-9-CM codes) presented an adjusted OR of an association with APS of 4.58 (95% confidence interval, 2.00–10.51).[42] Older studies reported IUGR to occur in approximately one-third of patients diagnosed with APS,[45,50] and aCL antibodies are significantly associated with IUGR as well.[38,51] Because IUGR is most commonly seen in the presence of preeclampsia, causality is difficult to establish.

Although there are no prospective trials studying the association between abruptio placenta and APS, Alfirevic and colleagues[39] noted an association between abruptio and aCL IgG antibodies in a systematic review in 2002.

Obstetric complications abound in the presence of APS, but therapeutic recommendations are either incomplete or inadequate. However, results from European registries of infants born to mothers with APS seem to fare well with no cases of neonatal thrombosis[52] and rare long-term complications. It is hoped that advances in understanding of the pathophysiology of APS will lead to more successful management schemes and therapy.

PATHOPHYSIOLOGY OF APS

The diagnosis of APS requires both the presence of aPL and specific clinical manifestations, including RPL, fetal demise, and obstetric complications such as preeclampsia and IUGR. The presence of aPL is the most common autoimmune risk factor for a treatable cause of RPL, fetal demise, and early, severe preeclampsia.[53,54] The presence of aPL is not simply diagnostic in obstetric APS, it is also pathogenic. Animal studies have indicated that the passive transfer of aPL promotes fetal loss and placental thrombosis, and also inhibits trophoblast and decidual cell functions in vitro.[55–57] Cross-species investigations have shown that the exposure of pregnant rats to a purified IgG fraction from women with APS directly inhibits embryo growth.[58] Histologic studies on the placentas from aPL-treated mice showed thrombotic lesions of decidua basalis maternal blood vessels and necrosis of the placental tissues. aPLs interact with phospholipid-binding plasma proteins to cause arterial and/or venous thrombosis in the absence of other conditions that promote blood coagulation. The two most clinically relevant phospholipid-binding proteins that react with aPL autoantibodies are β2GP1 and prothrombin.[53] aPLs impair fetal growth and development via mechanisms of thrombosis, inhibition of normal placentation, and local inflammatory destruction.

Thrombosis and aPLs

The primary hypothesis for the major pathogenic mechanism for aPL-induced pregnancy loss and fetal growth restriction is placental thrombosis. Thrombosis of vessels causes placental infarction with resultant impairment of maternal-fetal nutrient and oxygen exchange. This hypothesis is supported by the finding of thrombosis and infarction in the placentas of women with APS who had miscarriages in the first and second trimesters.[1,59,60] The scientific plausibility for placental thrombosis as a cause of obstetric complications in APS is supported by the evidence that increasing aCL titers are correlated with an increased risk of peripheral thrombosis.[61,62] The presence of LAC seems to cause a higher risk of thrombosis than aCL.[63] IgG from the sera of LAC-positive patients increased thromboxane synthesis in placental explants compared with controls. This relative increase in thromboxane activity would produce a thrombophilic state.[64] Other studies have indicated that aPL could promote thrombosis by interfering with protein C activation[65] and diminishing antithrombin activity.[66]

A major target molecule for aPL binding seems to be β2GP1, which is present on the surface of trophoblastic cell membranes.[20,21] β2GP1 is a cationic plasma protein that is bound to phosphatidylserine (PS), which is exposed on the surface of trophoblastic cell membranes undergoing syncytial formation. Although the physiologic role of β2GP1 is unclear, the molecule seems to inhibit thrombosis by reducing the conversion of prothrombin to thrombin on platelets and inhibiting the activation of the intrinsic coagulation cascade.[22] Polyclonal IgG from the sera of patients with APS binds to β2GP1 on trophoblastic cells in culture with potential thrombogenic consequences.[3,67] However, observations in murine models and humans are not consistent with the obligate involvement of β2GP1 as a natural inhibitor of placental thrombosis in APS. Mice deficient in β2GP1 have smaller litter sizes and placental insufficiency but otherwise have similar reproductive outcomes compared with control mice.[68] In addition, individuals have been identified who are deficient in β2GP1 but do not show the clinical signs of APS.[69]

Another mechanism for aPL-mediated thrombosis may involve a disruption of the normal function of a plasma protein called annexin V.[70] The binding of cationic annexin V molecules to the anionic PL molecules on the surface of the trophoblastic membrane seems to prevent thrombosis by forming a protective protein coat. This protective coat might prevent the activation of the clotting cascade by blocking the binding of activated factor X and prothrombin. In vitro studies indicate that aPL could displace annexin V from the surface of endothelial and trophoblastic cells in culture, thus activating the clotting cascade. This mechanism is supported by the finding that women with aPLs have diminished annexin V binding to the surface of trophoblastic cells of the intervillous space compared with controls.[71]

Mechanisms besides placental vascular thrombosis are likely to play a role in the RPL and pregnancy complications associated with obstetric APS. Histopathologic studies have not always confirmed thrombosis in the placentas from women with obstetric APS.[7,72,73] Meta-analyses examining the association of aPLs with placental thrombosis have evaluated index women with systemic thrombosis who were subsequently tested for aPLs, potentially introducing selection bias into these investigations. There have been no large prospective studies of unselected patients whose aPL status was determined before objective documentation of thrombotic complications. As a result, the temporal association between aPLs and the subsequent development of placental thrombosis has not been definitively documented.[74]

Defective Placentation

Abnormalities of early trophoblast invasion caused by aPLs are a likely pathogenic mechanism in obstetric APS.[75] Experimental models indicate that aPLs can directly retard trophoblast invasiveness, impair trophoblastic cellular differentiation and maturation, and diminish human chorionic gonadotropin secretion.[3,76] The histologic abnormality most frequently observed in APS-associated early pregnancy loss was defective decidual endovascular trophoblast invasion, rather than intervillous thrombosis. Exposure of trophoblastic cell monolayers to aPLs resulted in an increased rate of programmed cell death (apoptosis) and inhibition of syncytial formation.[58,77] The sequential expression of cell adhesion molecules between trophoblastic and decidual cells is involved in trophoblastic invasion during normal placentation. Using an in vitro model of trophoblast invasion, it was recently reported that aPLs might affect placental invasion through an abnormal trophoblastic expression of integrins and cadherins.[78]

These findings provide supportive evidence that aPLs may be pathogenic in obstetric APS by directly impairing normal placentation via a mechanism independent of placental or decidual thrombosis.

Local Inflammatory Events

The maternal immune system is transformed during normal pregnancy to prevent immune rejection of the fetoplacental unit. Acute inflammatory responses generally promote adverse pregnancy outcome and chemokine mediators favor a profile of T helper cells type 2 (Th2) responses in early pregnancy which block acute immune rejection.[45] Complement-mediated immune attack is suppressed in normal pregnancies, resulting in viable delivery by complement inhibitory proteins expressed on trophoblast cells.[79] Studies in mice indicate that inhibition of complement C3 activation and deficiencies of C5 and C5a seem to protect against pregnancy loss and fetal growth restriction.[80,81]

The binding of aPL to trophoblast cell membranes promotes complement activation, specifically C3a and C5a, resulting in thrombosis and pregnancy loss.[82] Instigators of inflammatory tissue injury caused by complement activation include the chemokine tumor necrosis factor (TNF) alpha and the cytokine receptor, tissue factor (TF). Exposure of pregnant mice to aPL causes an increase in decidual TNF-α levels, putatively secondary to C5 activation.[83] In an APS mouse model, antibody-mediated reduction of TNF-α helped prevent fetal resorption.[84] Therefore, TNF-α is a likely mediator that links complement activation and aPL to placental inflammatory injury. Complement activation (C5a–C5aR) increases TF expression in neutrophils, which increase generation of reactive oxygen species thus providing a novel mechanism to explain fetal loss.[85] An additional mechanism whereby TF could promote placental injury in APS is its capacity to activate the coagulation pathway, leading to thrombosis.[86]

More evidence is required to confirm the role of complement-mediated pregnancy loss in women with APS. Histopathologic studies reveal that placental tissue from APS gestations show a clustering of inflammatory cells and macrophages around blood vessels compared with controls.[87] Other investigations have not consistently shown the presence of complement complex deposition in placental tissue from women with APS.[88] Important future work will help determine whether therapy that targets interruption of complement-mediated inflammatory injury will be effective in improving pregnancy outcome in women with APS.

Mechanism of Therapeutic Benefit of Heparin

The therapeutic benefit of heparin and aspirin in improving outcomes in women with obstetric APS has been presumed to relate to their anticoagulant properties. However, the efficacy of heparin in the management of obstetric APS is achieved at a dosage lower than is required to achieve clinical anticoagulation. Studies in the murine model indicate that anticoagulants such as hirudin and fondaparinux are ineffective in the treatment of aPL-induced pregnancy loss, despite having anticoagulant effects similar to heparin.[89] Several mechanisms have been identified that may explain the beneficial effects of heparin independently of its anticoagulant action.

Low-molecular-weight heparin (LMWH) directly impedes aPL binding to trophoblast cells and reinstates normal trophoblast invasiveness and differentiation hindered by aPL. Heparin also can potentially regulate apoptosis in placental explants by increasing levels of Bcl-2, an antiapoptotic protein.[90] Furthermore, heparins have been shown to prevent complement activation in vitro, an action that would protect normal placentation from inflammatory injury. Exposure of trophoblastic cells to LMWH results in an increase in matrix metalloproteinases in trophoblastic cells, an action that would promote trophoblastic invasiveness.[91] Heparin sulfate directly binds aPL, providing a novel and alternative mechanism for its therapeutic benefit in treating obstetric APS.[92,93]

Thus, heparin may prevent pregnancy complications in obstetric APS by inhibiting the binding of aPL to trophoblastic cell membranes, modulating trophoblast apoptosis, promoting trophoblast cell invasiveness, and reducing complement activation with the ensuing inflammatory response at the decidual-placental interface. All of these mechanisms are independent of heparin's known anticoagulant property in inhibiting thrombosis.

MANAGEMENT OF APS IN PREGNANCY
Overview of Proposed Treatments

Only 20% to 30% of patients with LAC and/or positive levels of aPL who have had unsuccessful previous pregnancies have a successful delivery without treatment.[16,47] Comparison of studies in the literature is unsatisfactory because of differences in study design, patient selection, and treatment regimens. There are few randomized clinical trials, and variations in study definitions affect tabulated outcomes. Pregnancy outcomes are not always defined. Women with low levels of aPL are included in some studies. Moreover, aPL assays performed in laboratories with inappropriate standardization or controls may further complicate interpretation of results.

Several treatments have been proposed, including a single low-dose aspirin per day (81 mg), aspirin and low-dose or high-dose prednisone, aspirin and unfractionated heparin, aspirin and LMWH, and intravenous immunoglobulin.[94] All treatments seem to improve the live birth rate; however, the combination of unfractionated heparin with low-dose aspirin seems to provide the highest success rates.[34,35,48,49] Aspirin is thought to improve outcome by selective inhibition of thromboxane production thus restoring the balance with prostaglandin. Concomitant use of prednisone and heparin is generally not recommended because this combination has not been shown to be better than either alone and may increase the risk of fractures. In a randomized trial comparing heparin and aspirin versus prednisone and aspirin, Cowchock and colleagues included a small group of 20 women with at least 2 early losses.[46] However, patients were not assigned to treatment until after the documentation of a fetal heartbeat, thus the outcome that showed that the treatments were equal in achieving a successful outcome has been questioned. However, treatment with corticosteroids was associated with increased neonatal morbidity (preterm delivery and low birth weight) and increased maternal morbidity (pregnancy-induced hypertension and gestational diabetes). A more recent prospective randomized clinical trial comparing prednisone and aspirin (100 mg/d) for women with autoantibodies and unexplained recurrent fetal loss showed no benefit in promoting live birth with prednisone and aspirin but an increase in prematurity.[47]

Unfractionated Heparin Compared with LMWH

In our prospective trial of aspirin alone versus aspirin and heparin, a group of well-characterized women with APS ($\geq$3 early RPLs), an otherwise negative evaluation, and positive aPL on 2 occasions were given different treatments.[95] The group treated with aspirin alone had a 44% live birth rate, whereas the group treated with subcutaneous heparin and aspirin had a 78% live birth rate (P<.05). The incidence of maternal complications was low and there were no significant differences in the birth weight, incidence of pregnancy- induced hypertension (PIH), gestational diabetes, or cesarean section.

Low-dose heparin is emerging as the treatment of choice for RPL associated with antiphospholipid syndrome.[15,27,34,39,49,92,95] Heparin treatment is generally initiated at 5000 to 7500 U twice a day when the pregnancy test is positive. It is important to obtain a baseline platelet count and partial thromboplastin time. Heparin treatment is associated with heparin-induced osteopenia at total daily doses of more than 15,000 international units (IU) per day which, combined with the normal osteoporosis associated during pregnancy, can be accompanied by increased bone loss. The heparinized pregnant patient should increase her intake of calcium to 600 mg orally twice a day along with vitamin D 400 IU twice daily to optimize absorption of calcium and to reduce the risk of osteopenia (**Box 4**). Heparin is also reported to be associated with thrombocytopenia. However, the incidence in populations of patients treated at our center at daily doses of less than 15,000 IU per day has been less than 1%. During pregnancy, the normal platelet count is more than 100,000/mL compared with the nonpregnant state, in which platelet counts are normally more than 150,000/mL. If counts were normal before conception and decreased dramatically during pregnancy, the heparin dosage should be reduced. It is important to instruct patients carefully on the proper administration of subcutaneous heparin to minimize complications. We use an intensive one-on-one teaching session with a nurse specialist before conception and have found that using this type of therapy reduces the stress level of patients.

The first prospective, randomized trial suggested that low-molecular-weight heparin may be an effective alternative to unfractionated heparin in the treatment of APS.[96] In a 2-centered, nonrandomized study, the use of aspirin 81 mg daily in combination with LMWH during pregnancy for the prevention of RPL in women with APS seemed to be as safe as unfractionated heparin plus aspirin.[97] Large, randomized trials are required to determine differences in outcome with LMWH and low-dose aspirin compared with

Box 4
Guidelines for prophylactic heparin plus aspirin treatment of patients with RPL without a history of thromboembolism but with APS

1. Baseline nonpregnant studies of aPLs, complete blood count with platelets, PT, PTT, and lupus anticoagulant should be obtained. aPL assay should be confirmed before pregnancy.

2. Aspirin 81 mg should be initiated before conception and discontinued 4 weeks before the expected delivery date. Aspirin 81 mg should be resumed postpartum and continued for life unless otherwise contraindicated or until better recommendations are available.

3. Subcutaneous heparin (5000 units every 12 hours) should be initiated when pregnancy is confirmed unless instructed otherwise. Patients who weigh more than 80 kg (175 pounds) should use heparin 7500 units every 12 hours. Platelets and PTT tests should be checked every week for 2 weeks initially, 1 week following any adjustment in dose, and each trimester throughout pregnancy to evaluate for heparin-induced thrombocytopenia (patients with prior thromboembolic events should be fully anticoagulated).

4. Calcium carbonate (1200–1500 mg) with vitamin D (800–1000 IU) should be taken daily in divided doses once a patient starts heparin to decrease the bone loss associated with pregnancy and heparin therapy.

5. The pregnancy should be documented by ultrasonography by 7 weeks for the detection of fetal heart motion. Further sonography may be performed at 18 to 20 weeks.

6. Antenatal testing should begin at 28 to 30 weeks, based on the possible increased risk of fetal growth restriction and stillbirth. This testing may include kick counts, nonstress tests, and/or serial biophysical profiles. Serial scans for growth rate may be indicated.

7. Heparin should be continued until the patient initiates spontaneous labor or until the night before any scheduled induction or operative delivery. One heparin dose may be skipped the night before amniocentesis. Heparin should be restarted postpartum at the lowest predelivery dosage and continued for 4 weeks (in those patients with previous thromboembolic events, full anticoagulation should continue for 6 weeks postpartum).

8. For prolonged deliveries and operative deliveries, the use of pneumatic sequential compression devices or hose should be considered until the patient is ambulatory.

9. If the patient is fully anticoagulated and delivery is emergent, 1% protamine sulfate can be administered intravenously over 10 minutes (2.5 mg protamine per 1000 U heparin, maximum 50 mg protamine) if coagulation indicators are increased.

10. Patients should not use estrogen-containing birth control pills for contraception. Aspirin 81 mg daily is advised until further recommendations become available. Patients who smoke should be advised to stop.

Data from Refs.[15,49,95]

---

treatment with unfractionated heparin combined with low-dose aspirin in this group of patients.

Antepartum Surveillance

Antepartum testing has been recommended, based on the increased risk for poor obstetric outcome. For women who have had only first-trimester losses, it is usual to perform serial ultrasonic assessments weekly until the patients have progressed beyond the point of their prior losses. If the patient had a prior second-trimester or third-trimester fetal loss, serial antepartum testing is recommended.[15] Antepartum assessment using daily fetal kick counts, twice weekly nonstress tests, or weekly biophysical profile has been suggested.

POSTPREGNANCY CONSIDERATIONS
Immediately Postpartum

Women who had a vaginal delivery should ambulate as soon as possible. Women who had a cesarean delivery should continue to use pneumatic compression stockings until they are fully ambulating. Aspirin 81 mg a day can be reinitiated if not contraindicated for other reasons. Authorities recommend that women should receive thromboprophylaxis postpartum for 4 to 6 weeks.[15] In general, this recommendation includes women with and without a prior history of thrombosis. Supplemental calcium should be continued as long as the patient is taking heparin. Breast-feeding is not contraindicated for women taking low-dose aspirin or prophylactic heparin.

Lifelong Consequences of APS

Women with APS have been diagnosed with an acquired autoimmune syndrome similar to SLE. Once the diagnosis is made with appropriate clinical criteria, this should be considered to be a diagnosis that they carry for life. For example, an individual with lupus may have an exacerbation and be severely disabled with multiple abnormal laboratory tests, but, after resolution, her symptoms and laboratory tests may normalize. Many physicians are confused when a patient with APS who previously had positive tests presents years later and the test results have returned to normal; however, in our opinion the patient should still be considered to have the diagnosis of APS. As such, we recommend that, once the diagnosis of APS is made, women should not use estrogen-containing oral contraceptive pills but should use progestin-only pills, barrier methods, or intrauterine devices.[15] They should similarly not use tobacco products and should maintain a normal weight. Any correctable risk factors for future thrombosis, such as increased cholesterol, should also be corrected. We agree with the recommendation that these women should use lifelong aspirin 81 mg per day unless it is contraindicated for other reasons.[98] In general, these individuals should live a healthy lifestyle.

SUMMARY

It is unclear at this time what treatment, if any, is required for women who do not meet all the criteria for diagnosis of APS but are known to have aPL. In some cases, these women were tested because of a prior false-positive test for syphilis with subsequent identification of aPL. Women undergoing in vitro fertilization (IVF) have been tested and found to have an increased incidence of aPL.[99] However, a summary of all published reports on studies of at least 100 patients indicates that positive aPL in patients undergoing IVF does not influence pregnancy rates.[99]

In women who have a diagnosis of APS, meeting both clinical and laboratory criteria, the chance for successful pregnancy is reduced. In these cases, treatment seems to be a clear option, particularly in the case of patients with prior thromboembolic events. Current clinical guidelines support the use of subcutaneous heparin and aspirin. This treatment should begin with a positive pregnancy test, continue throughout pregnancy, and extend postpartum.

ACKNOWLEDGMENTS

The authors would like to thank John T. Kutteh for his assistance in the preparation and submission of this article. His contributions are greatly appreciated, as he helped to facilitate the timely submission of this article.

REFERENCES

1. DeWolf F, Carreras LO, Moerman P, et al. Decidual vasculopathy and extensive placental infarction in a patient with repeated thromboembolic accidents, recurrent fetal loss, and a lupus anticoagulant. Am J Obstet Gynecol 1982;142: 829–34.
2. Adler RR, Ng AK, Rote NS. Monoclonal antiphosphatidylserine antibody inhibits intercellular fusion of the choriocarcinoma line, JAR. Biol Reprod 1995;53: 905–10.
3. Katsuragawa H, Kanzaki H, Inoue T, et al. Monoclonal antibody against phosphatidylserine inhibits in vitro human trophoblastic hormone production and invasion. Biol Reprod 1997;56:50–8.
4. Quenby S, Mountfield S, Cartwright JE, et al. Antiphospholipid antibodies prevent extravillous trophoblast differentiation. Fertil Steril 2005;83:691–8.
5. Rand JH. Molecular pathogenesis of the antiphospholipid syndrome. Circ Res 2002;11:29–37.
6. Out HJ, Kooijman CD, Bruinse HW, et al. Histopathological findings in placentae from patients with intrauterine fetal death and antiphospholipid antibodies. Eur J Obstet Gynecol Reprod Biol 1991;41:179–86.
7. Kutteh WH, Rote NS, Silver R. Antiphospholipid antibodies and reproduction: the antiphospholipid antibody syndrome. Am J Reprod Immunol 1999;41: 133–52.
8. Schust DJ, Hill JA. Recurrent pregnancy loss. Philadelphia: Lippincott Williams & Wilkins; 2002.
9. Rand JH. The antiphospholipid syndrome. Annu Rev Med 2003;54:409–24.
10. Lockshin MD. Antiphospholipid antibody. J Am Med Assoc 1997;277:1549–54.
11. Alarcón-Segovia D, Deleze M, Oria CV, et al. Antiphospholipid antibodies and the antiphospholipid syndrome in systemic lupus erythematosus. A prospective analysis of 500 consecutive patients. Medicine (Baltimore) 1989;68: 353–65.
12. Kutteh WH, Lyda EC, Abraham SM, et al. Association of anticardiolipin antibodies and pregnancy loss in women with systemic lupus erythematosus. Fertil Steril 1993;60:449–99.
13. Miyakis S, Lockshin MD, Atsumi T, et al. International consensus statement on an update of the classification criteria for definite antiphospholipid syndrome (APS). J Thromb Haemost 2006;4:295–306.
14. Harris EN. Syndrome of the black swan. Br J Rheumatol 1986;26:324–6.
15. Branch DW, Holmgren C, Goldberg JD. Antiphospholipid syndrome. American College of Obstetricians and Gynecologists Practice Bulletin Number 118. Obstet Gynecol 2012;120:1514–21.
16. Silver RM, Draper ML, Scott JR, et al. Clinical consequences of antiphospholipid antibodies: an historic cohort study. Obstet Gynecol 1994;83:372–7.
17. Martin BA, Branch DW, Rodgers GM. Sensitivity of the activated partial thromboplastin time, the dilute Russell's viper venom time, and the Kaolin clotting time for the detection of the lupus anticoagulant: a direct comparison using plasma dilutions. Blood Coagul Fibrinolysis 1996;7:31–8.
18. Pengo V, Tripodi A, Reber G, et al. Update on the guidelines for lupus anticoagulant detection. J Thromb Haemost 2009;7:1737–40.
19. Harris EW, Gharavi AE, Boey ML, et al. Anticardiolipin antibodies:detection by radioimmunoassay and association with thrombosis in systemic lupus erythematosus. Lancet 1983;2:1211–4.

20. Di Simone N, Meroni PL, Del Papa N, et al. Antiphospholipid antibodies affect trophoblast gonadotrophin secretion and invasiveness by binding directly and through adhered beta-2 glycoprotein-1. Arthritis Rheum 2000; 43:140–50.

21. McIntyre J. Immune recognition at the maternal-fetal interface: overview. Am J Reprod Immunol 1992;28:127–31.

22. Schousboe I, Rasmussen M. Synchronized inhibition of the phospholipid mediated autoactivation of factor XII in plasma by beta-2 glycoprotein-1 and anti-beta-2 glycoprotein-1. Thromb Haemost 1995;73:798–804.

23. Yetman DL, Kutteh WH. Antiphospholipid antibody panels and Recurrent Pregnancy Loss: Prevalence of anticardiolipin antibodies compared with other antiphospholipid antibodies. Fertil Steril 1996;66:540–6.

24. Franklin RD, Kutteh WH. Antiphospholipid antibodies (APA) and Recurrent Pregnancy Loss: Treating a unique APA positive population. Human Reprod 2002;17: 2981–5.

25. Benedetto C, Marozio L, Tavella AM, et al. Coagulation disorders in pregnancy: acquired and inherited thrombophilias. Ann N Y Acad Sci 2010;1205: 106–17.

26. Hatasaka HH. Recurrent miscarriage epidemiologic factors, definitions, and incidence. Clin Obstet Gynecol 1994;37:625–34.

27. The Practice Committee of the American Society for Reproductive Medicine. Evaluation and treatment of Recurrent Pregnancy Loss. Fertil Steril 2012;98: 1103–11.

28. Jaslow CR, Carney JL, Kutteh WH. Diagnostic factors identified in 1020 women with two verses three or more recurrent pregnancy losses. Fertil Steril 2010;93: 1234–43.

29. Allison J, Schust D. Recurrent first trimester pregnancy loss: revised definitions and novel causes. Curr Opin Endocrinol Diabetes Obes 2009;16:446–50.

30. Vinatier D, Dufour P, Cosson M, et al. Antiphospholipid syndrome and recurrent miscarriages. Eur J Obstet Gynecol Reprod Biol 2001;96:37–50.

31. Chaleur C, Galanaud JP, Alonso S, et al. Observational study of pregnant women with a previous spontaneous abortion before the 10th gestation week with and without antiphospholipid antibodies. J Thromb Haemost 2010;8: 699–706.

32. Oron G, Ben-Haroush A, Goldfarb R, et al. Contribution of the addition of anti-beta 2-glycoprotein to the classification of antiphospholipid syndrome in predicting adverse pregnancy outcome. J Matern Fetal Neonatal Med 2011;24: 606–9.

33. Abrahams V. Mechanisms of antiphospholipid antibody-associated pregnancy complications. Thromb Res 2009;124:521–5.

34. Ziakas PD, Pavlou M, Voulgarelis M. Heparin treatment in antiphospholipid syndrome with recurrent pregnancy loss: a systematic review and meta-analysis. Obstet Gynecol 2010;115:1256–62.

35. Hoppe B, Burmester GR, Dorner T. Heparin or aspirin or both in the treatment of recurrent abortions in women with antiphospholipid antibody (syndrome). Curr Opin Rheumatol 2011;23:299–304.

36. Backos M, Rai R, Baxter N, et al. Pregnancy complications in women with recurrent miscarriage associated with antiphospholipid antibodies treated with low dose aspirin and heparin. Br J Obstet Gynaecol 1999;106:102–7.

37. Branch DW, Khamashta MA. Antiphospholipid syndrome: obstetric diagnosis, management, and controversies. Obstet Gynecol 2003;101:1333–44.

38. Robertson L, Wu O, Langhorne P, et al, for The Thrombosis Risk and Economic Assessment of Thrombophilia Screening (TREATS) Study. Thrombophilia in pregnancy; a systematic review. Br J Haematol 2006;132:171–96.

39. Alfirevic Z, Roberts D, Martlew V. How strong is the association between maternal thrombophilia and adverse pregnancy outcome? A systematic review. Eur J Obstet Gynecol Reprod Biol 2002;101:6–14.

40. Ruffatti A, Tonello M, Cavazzana A, et al. Laboratory classification categories and pregnancy outcome in patients with primary antiphospholipid syndrome prescribed antithrombotic therapy. Thromb Res 2009;123:482–7.

41. Werner E, Lockwood C. Thrombophilias and stillbirth. Clin Obstet Gynecol 2010; 53:617–27.

42. Nodler J, Moolamalla S, Ledger E, et al. Elevated antiphospholipid antibody titers and adverse pregnancy outcomes: analysis of a population-based hospital dataset. BMC Pregnancy Childbirth 2009;9:11–8.

43. do Prado A, Piovesan D, Staub H, et al. Association of anticardiolipin antibodies with pre-eclampsia. Obstet Gynecol 2010;116:1433–43.

44. Heilmann L, Schorsch M, Hahn T, et al. Antiphospholipid syndrome and pre-eclampsia. Semin Thromb Hemost 2011;37:141–5.

45. Branch DW, Silver RM, Blackwell JL, et al. Outcome of treated pregnancies in women with antiphospholipid syndrome: an update of the Utah experience. Obstet Gynecol 1992;80:614–20.

46. Cowchock FS, Reece EA, Balaban D, et al. Repeated fetal losses associated with antiphospholipid antibodies: a collaborative randomized trial comparing prednisone with low-dose aspirin treatment. Am J Obstet Gynecol 1992;166: 1318–23.

47. Laskin CA, Bombardier C, Hannah ME, et al. Prednisone and aspirin in women with autoantibodies and unexplained recurrent fetal loss. N Engl J Med 1997; 337:148–53.

48. Kutteh WH, Ermel LD. A clinical trial for the treatment of antiphospholipid antibody associated recurrent pregnancy loss with lower dose heparin and aspirin. Am J Reprod Immunol 1996;35:402–7.

49. Empson M, Lassere M, Craig JC, et al. Recurrent pregnancy loss with antiphospholipid antibody: a systematic review of therapeutic trials. Obstet Gynecol 2002;99:135–44.

50. Lima F, Khamashta MA, Buchanan NM, et al. A study of sixty pregnancies in patients with the antiphospholipid syndrome. Clin Exp Rheumatol 1996;14:131–6.

51. Yasuda M, Takakuwa K, Tokunage A, et al. Prospective studies of the association between anticardiolipin antibody and outcome of pregnancy. Obstet Gynecol 1995;86:555–9.

52. Motta M, Lachassinne E, Boffa MC, et al. European registry of infants born to mothers with antiphospholipid syndrome: preliminary results. Minerva Pediatr 2010;62(3 Suppl 1):25–7.

53. Levine JS, Branch DW, Rauch J. The antiphospholipid syndrome. N Engl J Med 2002;346:752–63.

54. Tincani A, Balestrieri G, Danieli E, et al. Pregnancy complications of the antiphospholipid syndrome. Autoimmunity 2003;36:27–32.

55. Meroni PL, Riboldi P. Pathogenic mechanisms mediating antiphospholipid syndrome. Curr Opin Rheumatol 2001;13:377–82.

56. Branch D, Dudley DJ, Mitchell MD, et al. Immunoglobulin G fraction from patients with antiphospholipid antibodies caused fetal death in BALB/c mice: a model for autoimmune fetal loss. Am J Obstet Gynecol 1990;63:210–6.

57. Blank M, Cohen J, Toder V, et al. Induction of antiphospholipid syndrome in naive mice with mouse lupus monoclonal and human polyclonal anti-cardiolipin antibodies. Proc Natl Acad Sci U S A 2001;88:3069–73.
58. Ornoy A, Yacobi S, Matalon ST, et al. The effects of antiphospholipid antibodies obtained from women with SLE/APS and associated pregnancy loss on rat embryos and placental explants in culture. Lupus 2003;2:573–8.
59. Hanly JG, Gladman DD, Rose TH, et al. Lupus pregnancy. A prospective study of placental changes. Arthritis Rheum 1988;31:358–66.
60. Nayar R, Lage JM. Placental changes in a first trimester missed abortion in maternal systemic lupus erythematosus with antiphospholipid syndrome: a case report and review of literature. Hum Pathol 1996;27:201–6.
61. Turiel M, Sarzi-Puttini P, Peretti R, et al. Thrombotic risk factors in primary antiphospholipid syndrome: a 5-year prospective study. Stroke 2005;36:1490–4.
62. Gharavi AE, Pierangeli SS, Espinola RG, et al. Antiphospholipid antibodies induced in mice by immunization with a cytomegalovirus-derived peptide cause thrombosis and activation of endothelial cells in vivo. Arthritis Rheum 2002;46: 545–52.
63. Galli M, Luciani D, Bertolini G, et al. Lupus anticoagulants are stronger risk factors for thrombosis than anticardiolipin antibodies in the antiphospholipid syndrome: a systematic review of the literature. Blood 2003;101: 1827–32.
64. Peaceman AM, Rehnberg KA. The effect of immunoglobulin G fractions from patients with lupus anticoagulant on placental prostacyclin and thromboxane production. Am J Obstet Gynecol 1993;169:1403–6.
65. Cariou R, Tobelem G, Soria C, et al. Inhibition of protein C activation by endothelial cells in the presence of lupus anticoagulant. N Engl J Med 1986;314:1193–4.
66. Cosgriff TM, Martin BA. Low functional and high antigenic antithrombin III level in a patient with the lupus anticoagulant and recurrent thrombosis. Arthritis Rheum 1981;24:94–6.
67. Vogt E, Ng AK, Rote NS. A model for the antiphospholipid antibody syndrome: monoclonal antiphosphatidylserine antibody induces intrauterine growth restriction in mice. Am J Obstet Gynecol 1996;174:700–7.
68. Robertson SA, Roberts CT, van BE, et al. Effect of beta2-glycoprotein I null mutation on reproductive outcome and antiphospholipid antibody-mediated pregnancy pathology in mice. Mol Hum Reprod 2004;10:409–16.
69. Yasuda S, Tsutsumi A, Chiba H, et al. beta(2)-glycoprotein I deficiency: prevalence, genetic background and effects on plasma lipoprotein metabolism and hemostasis. Atherosclerosis 2000;152:337–46.
70. Rand JH, Wu XX, Quinn AS, et al. The annexin A5-mediated pathogenic mechanism in the antiphospholipid syndrome: role in pregnancy losses and thrombosis. Lupus 2010;19:460.
71. Rand JH, Wu XX, Andree HA, et al. Pregnancy loss in the antiphospholipid-antibody syndrome–a possible thrombogenic mechanism. N Engl J Med 1997;337:154–60.
72. Out HJ, Bruinse HW, Christians CM, et al. A prospective, controlled multicenter study of the obstetric risks of pregnant women with antiphospholipid antibodies. Br J Obstet Gynaecol 1992;167:26–32.
73. Salafia CM, Cowchock FS. Placental pathology and antiphospholipid antibodies: a descriptive study. Am J Perinatol 1997;14:435–41.

74. Greaves G, Cohen H, MacHin SJ, et al. Guidelines on the investigation and management of the antiphospholipid syndrome. Br J Haematol 2000;109:704–815.
75. Sebire NJ, Fox H, Backos M, et al. Defective endovascular trophoblast invasion in primary antiphospholipid antibody syndrome-associated early pregnancy failure. Hum Reprod 2002;17:1067–71.
76. Di Simone N, Caliandro D, Castiellani R, et al. Low-molecular weight heparin restores in-vitro trophoblast invasiveness and differentiation in presence of immunoglobulin G fractions obtained from patients with antiphospholipid syndrome. Hum Reprod 1999;14:489–95.
77. Sthoeger ZM, Mozes E, Tartakovsky B. Anti-cardiolipin antibodies induce pregnancy failure by impairing embryonic implantation. Proc Natl Acad Sci U S A 1993;90:6464–7.
78. Di Simone N, Castellani R, Calandro D, et al. Antiphospholipid antibodies regulate the expression of trophoblast cell adhesion molecules. Fertil Steril 2002;77: 805–11.
79. Tedesco F, Narchi G, Radillo O, et al. Susceptibility of human trophoblast to killing by human complement and the role of the complement regulatory proteins. J Immunol 1993;151:1562–70.
80. Girardi G, Berman J, Redecha P, et al. Complement C5a receptors and neutrophils mediate fetal injury in the antiphospholipid syndrome. J Clin Invest 2003; 112:1644–54.
81. Holers VM, Girardi G, Mo L, et al. Complement C3 activation is required for antiphospholipid antibody-induced fetal loss. J Exp Med 2002;195:211–20.
82. Salmon JE, Girardi G. The role of complement in the antiphospholipid syndrome. Curr Dir Autoimmun 2004;7:133–48.
83. Berman J, Girardi G, Salmon JE. TNF-alpha is a critical effector and a target for therapy in antiphospholipid antibody induced pregnancy loss. J Immunol 2005; 174:485–90.
84. Blank M, Krause I, Wildbaum G, et al. TNFα DNA vaccination prevents clinical manifestations of experimental antiphospholipid syndrome. Lupus 2003;12: 546–9.
85. Boles J, Mackman N. Role of tissue factor in thrombosis in antiphospholipid antibody syndrome. Lupus 2010;19:370.
86. Alijotas-Reig J, Vilardell-Tarres M. Is obstetric antiphospholipid syndrome a primary nonthrombotic, proinflammatory, complement-mediated disorder related to antiphospholipid antibodies? Obstet Gynecol Surv 2010;65:39–45.
87. Stone S, Pijnenborg R, Vercruysse L, et al. The placental bed in pregnancies complicated by primary antiphospholipid syndrome. Placenta 2006;27:457–67.
88. Cavazzana I, Nebuloni M, Cetin I, et al. Complement activation in antiphospholipid syndrome: a clue for an inflammatory process? J Autoimmun 2007;28:160–4.
89. Girardi G, Redecha P, Salmon JE. Heparin prevents antiphospholipid antibody-induced fetal loss by inhibiting complement activation. Nat Med 2004;10: 1222–6.
90. Di Simone N, Castellani R, Raschi E, et al. Anti-β-2 GPI antibodies affect Bcl-2 and Bax trophoblast expression without evidence of apoptosis. Ann N Y Acad Sci 2006;1069:364–76.
91. Di Simone N, Di Nicuolo F, Sarguinetti M, et al. Low-molecular weight heparin induces in vitro trophoblast invasiveness: role of matrix metalloproteinases and tissue inhibitors. Placenta 2007;28:298–304.

92. Ermel LD, Marshburn PB, Kutteh WH. Interaction of heparin with antiphospholipid antibodies (ASA) from the sera of women with recurrent pregnancy loss (RPL). Am J Reprod Immunol 1995;33:14–20.
93. Franklin RD, Kutteh WH. Effects of unfractionated and low molecular weight heparin on antiphospholipid anatibody binding in vitro. Obstet Gynecol 2003; 101:4555–62.
94. Stephenson MD, Houlihan E, Tsang P, et al. Concomitant use of IVIG for treatment of the antiphospholipid antibody syndrome (APS) when ASA and heparin results in at least one adverse pregnancy outcome. Lupus 2002; 11:694.
95. Kutteh WH. Antiphospholipid antibody-associated recurrent pregnancy loss: treatment with heparin and low dose aspirin is superior to low dose aspirin alone. Am J Obstet Gynecol 1996;174:1584–9.
96. Stephenson MD, Ballem PJ, Tsang P, et al. Treatment of antiphospholipid antibody syndrome (APS) in pregnancy: a randomized pilot trial comparing low molecular weight heparin to unfractionated heparin. J Obstet Gynaecol 2004; 26:729–34.
97. Noble LS, Kutteh WH, Lashey N, et al. Antiphospholipid antibodies associated with recurrent pregnancy loss: prospective, multicenter, controlled pilot study comparing treatment with low-molecular-weight heparin versus unfractionated heparin. Fertil Steril 2005;83:684–90.
98. Erkan D, Merrill JT, Yazici Y, et al. High thrombosis rate after fetal loss in antiphospholipid syndrome: effective prophylaxis with aspirin. Arthritis Rheum 2001;44:1466–7.
99. Hornstein MD. Antiphospholipid antibodies in patients undergoing IVF: the data do not support testing. Fertil Steril 2000;74(4):635–6.

Inherited Thrombophilias and Adverse Pregnancy Outcomes
A Review of Screening Patterns and Recommendations

William B. Davenport, MD[a], William H. Kutteh, MD, PhD, HCLD[b],*

KEYWORDS

- Pregnancy • Inherited thrombophilias • Recurrent pregnancy loss • Preeclampsia
- Intrauterine growth restriction • Placental abruption • OB/GYN

KEY POINTS

- Historically, much controversy has existed regarding the association of inherited thrombophilias with adverse pregnancy outcomes.
- The current guidelines do not recommend screening unless a personal or strong family history of venous thromboembolism is present, but the authors' survey of physician screening patterns has suggested that up to 40% of physicians may screen contrary to the current guidelines.
- Over 90% of both general Obstetrician/Gynecologists and Reproductive Endocrinologists are appropriately testing patients with recurrent pregnancy loss for anticardiolipin antibodies and the lupus anticoagulant with the overwhelming majority using indicated treatment during pregnancy.
- This article summarizes the existing evidence for each inherited thrombophilia and reviews the current guidelines.

INTRODUCTION

Three decades ago, antiphospholipid antibodies (aPL) were proposed to have a causal association with recurrent pregnancy loss (RPL), suspected because of placental clots that were observed after pregnancy loss with subsequent positive serum aPLs. Following the hypothesis-inducing investigations, an association was found between aPL and RPL. However, it was not until 1996 that Kutteh and

The authors have nothing to disclose.
[a] Department of Obstetrics and Gynecology, University of Vermont, 89 Beaumont Avenue, Given C262, Burlington, VT 05406, USA; [b] Department of Obstetrics and Gynecology, Vanderbilt University Medical Center, Fertility Associates of Memphis, 80 Humphreys Center, Suite 307, Memphis, TN 38120, USA
* Corresponding author.
E-mail address: wkutteh@fertilitymemphis.com

Obstet Gynecol Clin N Am 41 (2014) 133–144
http://dx.doi.org/10.1016/j.ogc.2013.10.005
0889-8545/14/$ – see front matter © 2014 Elsevier Inc. All rights reserved.

colleagues[1] found that treatment of pregnant women who have aPL syndrome with heparin and aspirin increased the live birth rate to 80%.[2]

With a causal role of aPL established, research was driven by further hypotheses that inherited thrombophilias may cause pregnancy losses via their resulting hypercoagulability and expanded to also include other adverse pregnancy outcomes, including the effects on preeclampsia, intrauterine growth restriction (IUGR), placental abruption, and stillbirth. The various case control trials that resulted have yielded conflicting conclusions regarding inherited thrombophilias and adverse pregnancy outcomes, and randomized controlled trials are lacking. No causal role has been established to date.[3] The authors' group performed a survey of the screening and treatment patterns for thrombophilia in pregnancy among obstetricians (OBs) and reproductive endocrinologists (REIs) regarding thrombophilias in pregnancy. The authors found that many physicians may still screen and treat for inherited thrombophilias beyond the recommendations. This article provides an overview of the pathophysiology of the most common inherited thrombophilias and historical findings of their relationships to adverse pregnancy outcomes. It also summarizes the current recommendations for screening and treatment of inherited thrombophilias and presents recent practice patterns of physicians in response to this evidence.

OVERVIEW

Inherited thrombophilia is defined as a genetic predisposition to venous thromboembolism (VTE), usually a genetic deletion or alteration of a functional protein in the coagulation cascade. The most common inherited thrombophilias include factor V Leiden (FVL G1691A) mutation, prothrombin gene mutation (prothrombin G20210A), protein C deficiency (PCD), protein S deficiency (PSD), methyltetrahydrofolate reductase (MTHFR) mutation, and antithrombin III (AT) deficiency. Each of these has a common role in inducing a hypercoagulable state via direct or indirect augmentation of prothrombin to thrombin, its active clot-inducing form (**Fig. 1**). Because hypercoagulability with inherited thrombophilias has been well established, screening of pregnant women with a personal history of VTE has been generally well accepted in practice, with the purpose of providing thromboembolic prophylaxis if needed. This practice is supported by the most recent guidelines, and its acceptance is confirmed in the authors' survey findings of physicians' practices.[4] Screening in the presence of a family history of VTE has also been historically accepted but has recently been challenged as not being founded on evidence.[4–9] Subsequently, the practice is currently being reassessed, with some evidence against screening in women with a positive family history of VTE.[9]

A larger controversy has existed in the recent past around the utility of screening for inherited thrombophilias in women with a history of adverse pregnancy outcome or loss. Several strong arguments exist against screening in this population. Perhaps most importantly, only weak associations have been found between hypercoagulability and pregnancy outcomes; no causative relationship has been established.[3] Even more, many inherited thrombophilias are common in the general population, and most of these women have normal pregnancy outcomes.[10] From the standpoint of thromboembolism prevention, some argue that inherited genetic aberrations in clotting proteins are less likely to be significant in the absence of a thromboembolic event history and that screening this population is akin to screening the general population, which has shown to be cost-ineffective.[11] Because of these positions, recommendations are against screening women in this group.

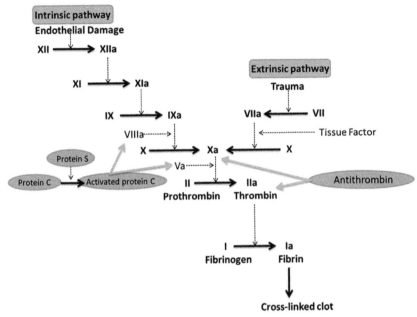

Fig. 1. Cascade of thrombus formation.

Despite the aforementioned arguments and published recommendations regarding the utility of screening in pregnant women with a history of loss or adverse outcomes, the authors' findings have suggested that many physicians continue to screen this population. These convictions are not unfounded, and several historical studies support this stance. Most studies in support of this practice hypothesize microthrombi, thrombosis, and infarction of the placenta as contributing causes of pregnancy complications or loss.[1,11,12] In addition, an argument exists that women with any type of thromboembolic defect have a higher prevalence of pregnancy complications.[13] Following is a summary of the available evidence regarding each inherited thrombophilia in relation to adverse pregnancy outcomes and the risk of VTE. All data reported here are assuming an absence of personal or family history of VTE.

Factor V Leiden

Activated factor V is a clotting protein that works in conjunction with activated factor X to directly convert prothrombin to thrombin. A specific mutant form of this protein, factor V Leiden (F5 c.1691G>A and p.Arg506Gln), is resistant to inactivation, leading to higher amounts of activated factor V, more thrombin formation, and, thus, a hypercoagulable state (see **Fig. 1**). Although its heterozygous form is the most common inherited thrombophilia, its prevalence is still low in the general population.[4] Less than 0.3% of these heterozygotes will have a VTE in pregnancy.[4]

Concerning adverse fetal outcomes, 2 recent comprehensive reviews of the literature have determined that carriers of FVL G1691A have an increased relative risk for RPL (odds ratio [OR] 1.52, 95% confidence interval [CI] 1.06–2.19 and OR 2.02, 95% CI 1.60–2.55).[14,15] However, the maternal-fetal medicine (MFM) network also emphasized a low absolute risk (4.2%) of pregnancy loss in women with FVL G1691A.[15] No significant association exists between FVL G1691A and preeclampsia or small gestational age.[15,16] Associations between placental abruption and FVL G1691A are also lacking.[17–19] However, a more recent MFM network case control study, although confirming a lack of association with placental abruption, did find an increase in fetal hypoxia-inducing factors in the placentas of mothers with FVL G1691A compared with age-matched controls.[20] The current guidelines agree that evidence is inadequate to recommend screening for factor V Leiden in women with adverse pregnancy outcomes of any kind.[4,9,11,14]

Prothrombin

Prothrombin G20210A substitution mutation (F2 c.20210G>A) is the second most common inherited thrombophilia, second only to heterozygous factor V Leiden. A mutated form causes a deficiency in thrombin, with a resulting increase in the concentration of prothrombin in the plasma (see **Fig. 1**). VTE incidence with prothrombin G20210A is low, with one early study suggesting prothrombin G20210A heterozygotes to have an absolute risk of less than 0.5% and homozygotes to only reach 2% to 3%. Concerning RPL, Bradley's[14] comprehensive literature review suggested that women with this mutation were overall twice as likely to have RPL as those without the prothrombin G20210A mutation (OR 2.07, 95% CI 1.59–2.7), but the MFM network determined no association in their case control study and meta analysis.[14,15,21] Both literature reviews stated that no definitive conclusion could be made about RPL and prothrombin G20210A because of a paucity of studies. There is consensus among all published reviews of literature that no association exists between prothrombin G20210A and preeclampsia or small for gestational age (SGA).[15,16,22] One study has suggested a correlation with placental abruption, but most have found no correlation between prothrombin G20210A and placental abruption.[16,21,23] Accordingly, the American Congress of Obstetricians and Gynecologists (ACOG) recommends against screening for prothrombin G20210A in women with any history of adverse pregnancy outcomes.[4]

Protein C Deficiency and Protein S Deficiency

Protein S and activated protein C, in combination, are necessary for the activation of factors V and VIII, as summarized in **Fig. 1**. Therefore, a deficiency in either of these proteins can result in a hypercoagulable state. Although the risk of VTE during pregnancy with either protein deficiency is up to 7% in the presence of a personal or family history of VTE, the absolute risk of VTE in the absence of such history is 0.1% and 0.1% to 0.8%, respectively.[4] Further, the prevalence of the disorders is only 0.2% to 0.3% in the general population. No studies have found an association between protein C Deficiency (PCD) or Protein S Deficiency (PSD) and early pregnancy loss, IUGR, or placental abruption. A review of literature from 2002 that included only 3 to 5 pertinent studies found an increased risk of preeclampsia with PCD (OR 21.5, CI 4.4–414.4) and PSD (OR 12.7, CI 4.0–39.7), with an absolute risk of 1.4% and 12.3%, respectively. The same study suggested an increase in stillbirth among those with PSD (OR 16.2, CI 5.0–52.3), with an absolute risk of 6%.[23] However, because of the small number of studies with relatively few participants, the ACOG currently does not recommend screening for PSD or PCD in women with any history of adverse pregnancy outcomes.[4]

Antithrombin Deficiency

Antithrombin is a small protein that inactivates both factor Xa and thrombin, and serves as a regulator of clot formation (see **Fig. 1**). A rare deficiency in this protein results in severe coagulopathy, increasing the risk up to 25 times those with normal antithrombin levels. Women with antithrombin III deficiency do indeed have an increased risk of embryonic demise and fetal death compared with the general population.[24–27] However, because of the low prevalence (1 out of 2500), screening is not recommended in those with a prior pregnancy loss. Studies observing its effects on other adverse pregnancy outcomes are lacking, also due to low prevalence.

Methylene Tetrahydrofolate Reductase

Methylene tetrahydrofolate reductase (MTHFR) is one of 3 enzymes that is essential for the metabolism of folic acid and is responsible for directly converting homocysteine to methionine. A mutation in this enzyme can cause increased levels of substrate homocysteine. Hyperhomocysteinemia debatably can result in a hypercoagulable state at the endothelium and has historically been associated with RPL[28]; but its relationship to thrombosis is only theoretical.[29] Two predominant mutations exist, MTHFR C677T and A1298C. Most recently, however, evidence has suggested that homocysteine is only a marker for thrombosis rather than a cause and that it must be combined with other thrombophilias to present any significant risk of VTE.[29–33] The existing data suggest an absence of any correlation with preeclampsia, IUGR, or placental abruption. However, the ACOG and the MFM network have determined that data are insufficient to determine the correlation.[20,22,34] Accordingly, the ACOG does not recommend screening women for MTHFR with any history of adverse fetal outcomes or with a history of VTE.[4]

MTHFR polymorphisms are also associated with an increased risk of neural tube defects (NTDs) because of low serum folic acid.[35] Women delivering a baby with an NTD have more than twice the incidence of having an MTHFR C677T polymorphism.[36] In addition, the combination of MTHFR C677T polymorphism with MTHFR A1298C polymorphism may further increase the risk of NTDs.[37] Therefore, the authors think it is prudent to treat these patients with amounts of folic acid similar to those used to treat patients who had a prior infant with an NTD.[36–38]

Combined Defects

Most studies have only observed VTE risks on pregnancy outcomes with individual thrombophilias. However, a few have assessed combinations of these disorders, such as FVL G1691A/prothrombin G20210A double heterozygosity and FVL G1691A in the presence of an MTHFR mutation, concluding that an additive or synergistic effect is present.[26,39–44] This distinction should be made, although further exploration of this topic is beyond the scope of this review.

Acquired Thrombophilias

Because of their nongenetic preponderance, acquired thrombophilias are classified separately from inherited thrombophilias and are summarized only briefly for the purpose of contrast because these disorders are also beyond the scope of this review. The most common acquired thrombophilia involves the presence of aPL. The presence of these antibodies has been associated with second-trimester as well as first-trimester pregnancy loss.[45,46] Therefore, it is recommended to screen for the most common of these antibodies (lupus anticoagulant, anticardiolipin, and anti-beta2 glycoprotein) in women with a history of more than 2 or 3 first-trimester losses and in women with one or more loss after 20 weeks with no alternative explanation.[4,11] It is also well established that treating these thrombophilias with heparin and aspirin improves pregnancy outcomes.[1,2]

TREATMENT OF INHERITED THROMBOPHILIAS

Given the current lack of evidence to support an association between adverse pregnancy outcomes and inherited thrombophilias, it is currently not recommended to treat inherited thrombophilias with adverse pregnancy outcomes alone in mind.[4] However, treatment is justifiable in some patients with known thrombophilias who are at an increased risk of VTE during pregnancy.[47] The ACOG's treatment recommendations have been abbreviated and summarized in **Table 1**. They specifically address thresholds at which to begin anticoagulants, which can be used to treat all known inherited thrombophilias except MTHFR mutations. The guidelines do not address the treatment of known MTHFR mutations for VTE prevention, but the traditional treatment has been vitamin B and folate. However, evidence now suggests that vitamin B supplementation does not reduce VTE incidence.[32,48] Therefore, if one decides to treat these mutations, folate alone may be the best choice.

Table 1
Recommended thromboprophylaxis for pregnancies complicated by inherited thrombophilias

Clinical Scenario	Antepartum Management	Postpartum Management
Low-risk thrombophilia[a] without previous VTE	Surveillance only or prophylactic heparin	Surveillance only if no risk factors; postpartum anticoagulation if risks factors[b]
Low-risk thrombophilia[a] with a single previous episode of VTE; not receiving long-term anticoagulation therapy	Surveillance only or prophylactic heparin	Postpartum anticoagulation therapeutic or intermediate-dose heparin
High-risk thrombophilia[c] without previous VTE	Prophylactic heparin	Postpartum anticoagulation therapy
High-risk thrombophilia[c] with a single previous episode of VTE; not receiving long-term anticoagulation therapy	Prophylactic, intermediate-dose or adjusted-dose heparin	Postpartum anticoagulation therapy or intermediate- or adjusted-dose heparin
Thrombophilia or no thrombophilia with 2 or more episodes of VTE; not receiving long-term anticoagulation therapy	Prophylactic or therapeutic-dose heparin	Postpartum anticoagulation therapy or therapeutic-dose heparin for 6 wk
Thrombophilia or no thrombophilia with 2 or more episodes of VTE; receiving long-term anticoagulation therapy	Therapeutic-dose heparin	Resumption of long-term anticoagulation therapy

[a] Low-risk thrombophilia: factor V Leiden heterozygous; prothrombin G20210A heterozygous; PCD or PSD.
[b] First-degree relative with a history of a thrombotic episode before 50 years of age or other major thrombotic risk factors (eg, obesity, prolonged immobility).
[c] High-risk thrombophilia: antithrombin deficiency; double heterozygous for prothrombin G20210A mutation and factor V Leiden; factor V Leiden homozygous or prothrombin G20210A mutation homozygous.
Adapted from James A. Practice bulletin no. 123: thromboembolism in pregnancy. Obstet Gynecol 2011;118(3):718–29; with permission.

PHYSICIAN PRACTICE PATTERNS

The authors' group distributed questionnaires regarding screening patterns of physicians for thrombophilia in pregnant women. Surveys were given to physicians only and were distributed at the beginning of 4 national meetings to OBs and REIs. The survey explored the clinical scenarios in which each physician would screen for thrombophilias, which tests they routinely ordered once the decision to order an evaluation had been made, and the treatment modalities used after an abnormal test result. Participants were given the survey before the meeting and were asked to respond to the survey based on their current practice pattern. Response rates at individual meetings ranged from 76% to 87% and were not considered significantly different between meetings. A total of 186 surveys were evaluated.

Thrombophilia Testing Criteria

Almost all physicians (97%) reported that a personal history of thrombosis warranted screening, and slightly fewer reported screening in patients with a family history of thrombosis (82%) (**Table 2**). Most physicians (90%) reported testing a patient with an unexplained fetal death at more than 20 weeks' gestation, but still 46% said they would screen a patient with a single loss at less than 20 weeks' gestation. Most physicians (94%) considered women with a history of 3 or more recurrent first-trimester miscarriages to be candidates for a thrombophilia evaluation, and 76% indicated that they offered testing after 2 early losses. Several physicians reported screening patients based on the fetal outcome of a prior abruption, with 62% screening patients if the abruption resulted in fetal demise compared with 37% if it resulted in a live birth; 42% screened a patient with a prior IUGR baby. Only a minority of REIs reported screening for assisted reproductive technology, whether it was a new patient (2%)

| Table 2 | | | | |
| Candidates for thrombophilia evaluation | | | | |
	ALL MDs[a] (%)	OB/GYN (%)	REI (%)	P
≥3 RPL	173/185 (94)	72/77 (94)	101/108 (94)	.57
≥2 RPL	141/185 (76)	55/77 (71)	86/108 (80)	.13
ART failed attempt	29/104 (28)	N/A	29/104 (28)	—
ART new attempt	2/102 (2)	N/A	2/102 (2)	—
Personal history thrombosis	181/186 (97)	75/78 (96)	106/108 (98)	.44
Family history thrombosis	150/183 (82)	61/77 (79)	89/106 (84)	.59
Stillbirth or IUFD >20 wk	164/183 (90)	66/78 (85)	98/105 (93)	.35
Spontaneous pregnancy loss[b]	81/176 (46)	31/76 (41)	50/100 (50)	.72
Prior IUGR	76/181 (42)	33/77 (43)	43/104 (41)	.64
Abruption, demise	112/181 (62)	50/75 (67)	62/106 (58)	.69
Abruption, live birth	65/177 (37)	27/73 (37)	38/104 (37)	.59
Personal history thrombophilia	161/183 (88)	63/77 (82)	98/106 (92)	.06
Prior baby with NTD	32/182 (18)	7/76 (9)	25/106 (24)	.01[c]
Sister with baby with NTD	23/181 (13)	5/76 (7)	18/105 (17)	.03[c]

Abbreviations: ART, assisted reproductive technology; GYN, gynecologist; IUFD, intrauterine fetal demise; N/A, not applicable.
 [a] Not all participants answered all survey questions, so the numbers are not equal to the total number of respondents.
 [b] Spontaneous pregnancy loss defined as less than 20 weeks.
 [c] Significantly different results between OB/GYNs and REIs.

or a previously failed cycle (28%) (see **Table 2**). There were no significant differences among specialties in testing criteria except that significantly more REIs offered screening for a personal or family history of NTDs than did OBs.

Thrombophilia Tests Used

When assessing which thrombophilia tests were routinely ordered in each physician's thrombophilia evaluation, almost all participants reported ordering anticardiolipin antibodies (98%) and lupus anticoagulant (97%) (**Table 3**). Most physicians included DNA testing for prothrombin G20210A (76%) and FVL G1691A mutations (90%) with no difference between specialties. Significantly more REIs reported screening for PCD (75% vs 53%; $P<.01$), PSD (73% vs 55%; $P<.01$), and AT deficiency (60% vs 42%; $P = .01$) (data not shown). More than a third of all physicians reported testing for polymorphisms on MTHFR (see **Table 3**).

Thrombophilia Treatment Patterns

The final section of the authors' survey examined which thrombophilias each physician treated and the treatment modality of each. Most REIs and generalists (80%–90%) reported treating patients who had an acquired thrombophilia, homozygous factor V Leiden, PCD, or PSD and treated homozygous and heterozygous disorders with equal frequency between specialties. However, more REIs treated an abnormal random homocysteine level in pregnancy than did OB/GYNs (80% vs 45%, $P<.01$) (data not shown). Concerning treatment modalities, most treated aPL, prothrombin G20210A, PCD, PSD, and AT with heparin, either alone or in combination with aspirin (**Table 4**).

DISCUSSION

The authors assessed how actual reported treatment patterns compared with the current guidelines by the ACOG. As expected, most of the practice patterns need no modification in order to remain in compliance with the most recent recommendations.[4,11] However, several practice patterns varied from the most recent guidelines. As detailed earlier, the ACOG's most recent recommendations hold that evidence is insufficient to screen for thrombophilias based on previous adverse pregnancy outcomes (IUGR, stillbirth, abruption, or pregnancy loss) alone in the absence of additional risk factors for thrombosis.[4] However, around 40% of physicians treated these women, suggesting that many are still following older literature, which suggests that inherited thrombophilias are associated with adverse pregnancy outcomes.

Table 3
Thrombophilia testing routinely being ordered by physicians

	ALL MDs[a] (%)	OB/GYN (%)	REI (%)	P
Anticardiolipin antibody	181/185 (98)	75/78 (96)	106/107 (99)	.72
Lupus anticoagulant antibody	180/186 (97)	74/78 (95)	106/108 (98)	.25
Antiphospholipid panel	147/183 (80)	67/78 (86)	80/105 (76)	.02[b]
Factor V Leiden G1691A	166/185 (90)	71/78 (91)	95/107 (89)	.41
Activated protein C resistance	98/182 (54)	33/77 (43)	65/105 (62)	.04[b]
Prothrombin G20210A	140/184 (76)	53/77 (69)	87/107 (81)	.07
MTHFR	75/178 (42)	20/73 (27)	56/105 (53)	<.01[b]

[a] Not all participants answered all survey questions, so the numbers are not equal to the total number of respondents.
[b] Significantly different results between OB/GYNs and REIs.

Table 4
Treatment patterns for thrombophilias (all physicians)[a]

	n[b]	Heparin[c] and/or Aspirin		Aspirin Only		Vitamin B and/or Folic Acid	
Anticardiolipin antibody	135	109	81%	19	14%	8	6%
Lupus anticoagulant antibody	128	107	84%	16	13%	7	5%
Antiphospholipid panel	107	86	81%	14	13%	8	7%
Factor V Leiden	121	108	89%	3	2%	8	7%
Activated protein C resistance	52	41	79%	5	10%	7	13%
Prothrombin mutation	78	70	90%	5	6%	4	5%
MTHFR C677T	61	12	20%	1	2%	59	97%
PCD	71	59	83%	8	11%	6	8%
PSD	67	54	81%	7	10%	7	10%
Antithrombin deficiency	47	41	87%	1	2%	4	9%
Anti-B2 glycoprotein	18	13	72%	2	11%	3	18%
Hyperhomocysteinemia	51	5	10%	1	2%	37	73%

[a] The numerator is equal to the number of physicians who treated the patient with the indicated treatment modality, and the denominator is equal to the number of physicians who both treated the indicated thrombophilia and answered the question concerning treatment modality. Not all participants answered all survey questions, so the numbers are not equal to the total number of respondents.
[b] Not all participants answered all survey questions, so the numbers are not equal to total number of respondents.
[c] Heparin includes both low-molecular-weight heparin and unfractionated heparin in either prophylactic or therapeutic doses.

Nevertheless, the authors agree that evidence is not adequate to make a definitive association between these pregnancy outcomes and inherited thrombophilias.

For those who meet the appropriate criteria for inherited thrombophilia screening, the ACOG recommends that the following tests be ordered: factor V Leiden, prothrombin G20210A, protein C and S, and antithrombin III.[4] Most physicians currently order all of the aforementioned tests; but greater than 40% of physicians reported also ordering MTHFR and homocysteine levels in their thrombophilia screen, both of which are not considered part of the recommended thrombophilia evaluation according to the ACOG. However, some of these decisions may have been based on the well-supported association of MTHFR polymorphisms with NTDs.[36–38]

Concerning treatment, the ACOG recommends that only acquired thrombophilias be treated for RPL and then with heparin and aspirin. Although more than half of the physicians appropriately treat these antibodies, a large percentage still only use heparin or aspirin, which has been shown to be inferior to combination therapy.[1,2] Most of the physicians who treat inherited thrombophilias appropriately use heparin with or without aspirin (see **Table 4**).

SUMMARY OF CURRENT STATE OF RESEARCH AND FUTURE DIRECTION

Overall, discrepancies in the literature do still exist concerning appropriate screening and management of those with prior adverse pregnancy outcomes. Large prospective, multicentered trials and evaluation of national databases, which are currently being conducted, will be required to clearly determine the risks associated with inherited thrombophilias in this regard. Until these data are available, physicians should compare their current practice patterns for thrombophilia screening with the guidelines in the ACOG practice bulletin, with an emphasis on individualizing their management when the data are not sufficient.

REFERENCES

1. Kutteh WH. Antiphospholipid antibody-associated recurrent pregnancy loss: treatment with heparin and low-dose aspirin is superior to low-dose aspirin alone. Am J Obstet Gynecol 1996;174(5):1584–9.
2. Rai R, Cohen H, Dave M, et al. Randomised controlled trial of aspirin and aspirin plus heparin in pregnant women with recurrent miscarriage associated with phospholipid antibodies (or antiphospholipid antibodies). BMJ 1997;314(7076):253–7.
3. Rodger MA, Paidas M, Mclintock C, et al. Inherited thrombophilia and pregnancy complications revisited. Obstet Gynecol 2008;112(2 Pt 1):320–4.
4. Lockwood C, Wendel G. Practice bulletin no. 124: inherited thrombophilias in pregnancy. Obstet Gynecol 2011;118(3):730–40.
5. van Sluis GL, Sohne M, El Kheir DY, et al. Family history and inherited thrombophilia. J Thromb Haemost 2006;4(10):2182–7.
6. Wichers IM, Tanck MW, Meijers JC, et al. Assessment of coagulation and fibrinolysis in families with unexplained thrombophilia. Thromb Haemost 2009;101(3): 465–70.
7. Villani M, Tiscia GL, Margaglione M, et al. Risk of obstetric and thromboembolic complications in family members of women with previous adverse obstetric outcomes carrying common inherited thrombophilias. J Thromb Haemost 2012; 10(2):223–8.
8. Lussana F, Coppens M, Cattaneo M, et al. Pregnancy-related venous thromboembolism: risk and the effect of thromboprophylaxis. Thromb Res 2012;129(6): 673–80.
9. Horton AL, Momirova V, Dizon-Townson D, et al. Family history of venous thromboembolism and identifying factor V Leiden carriers during pregnancy. Obstet Gynecol 2010;115(3):521–5.
10. Branch DW. The truth about inherited thrombophilias and pregnancy. Obstet Gynecol 2010;115(1):2–4.
11. Bates SM, Greer IA, Pabinger I, et al. Venous thromboembolism, thrombophilia, antithrombotic therapy, and pregnancy: American College of Chest Physicians evidence-based clinical practice guidelines (8th edition). Chest 2008; 133(Suppl 6):844S–86S.
12. Dizon-Townson DS, Meline L, Nelson LM, et al. Fetal carriers of the factor V Leiden mutation are prone to miscarriage and placental infarction. Am J Obstet Gynecol 1997;177(2):402–5.
13. Rey E, Kahn SR, David M, et al. Thrombophilic disorders and fetal loss: a meta-analysis. Lancet 2003;361(9361):901–8.
14. Bradley LA, Palomaki GE, Bienstock J, et al. Can factor V Leiden and prothrombin G20210A testing in women with recurrent pregnancy loss result in improved pregnancy outcomes?: results from a targeted evidence-based review. Genet Med 2012;14(1):39–50.
15. Rodger MA, Betancourt MT, Clark P, et al. The association of factor V Leiden and prothrombin gene mutation and placenta-mediated pregnancy complications: a systematic review and meta-analysis of prospective cohort studies. PLoS Med 2010;7(6):e1000292.

16. Howley HE, Walker M, Rodger MA. A systematic review of the association between factor V Leiden or prothrombin gene variant and intrauterine growth restriction. Am J Obstet Gynecol 2005;192(3):694–708.
17. Dizon-Townson D, Miller C, Sibai B, et al. The relationship of the factor V Leiden mutation and pregnancy outcomes for mother and fetus. Obstet Gynecol 2005;106(3):517–24.
18. Jaaskelainen E, Toivonen S, Romppanen EL, et al. M385T polymorphism in the factor V gene, but not Leiden mutation, is associated with placental abruption in Finnish women. Placenta 2004;25(8–9):730–4.
19. Prochazka M, Happach C, Marsal K, et al. Factor V Leiden in pregnancies complicated by placental abruption. BJOG 2003;110(5):462–6.
20. Rogers BB, Momirova V, Dizon-Townson D, et al. Avascular villi, increased syncytial knots, and hypervascular villi are associated with pregnancies complicated by factor V Leiden mutation. Pediatr Dev Pathol 2010;13(5):341–7.
21. Silver RM, Zhao Y, Spong CY, et al. Prothrombin gene G20210A mutation and obstetric complications. Obstet Gynecol 2010;115(1):14–20.
22. Infante-Rivard C, Rivard GE, Yotov WV, et al. Absence of association of thrombophilia polymorphisms with intrauterine growth restriction. N Engl J Med 2002;347(1):19–25.
23. Alfirevic Z, Roberts D, Martlew V. How strong is the association between maternal thrombophilia and adverse pregnancy outcome? A systematic review. Eur J Obstet Gynecol Reprod Biol 2002;101(1):6–14.
24. Di Nisio M, Middeldorp S, Buller HR. Direct thrombin inhibitors. N Engl J Med 2005;353(10):1028–40.
25. Blumenfeld Z, Brenner B. Thrombophilia-associated pregnancy wastage. Fertil Steril 1999;72(5):765–74.
26. Preston FE, Rosendaal FR, Walker ID, et al. Increased fetal loss in women with heritable thrombophilia. Lancet 1996;348(9032):913–6.
27. Sanson BJ, Friederich PW, Simioni P, et al. The risk of abortion and stillbirth in antithrombin-, protein C-, and protein S-deficient women. Thromb Haemost 1996;75(3):387–8.
28. Peng F, Labelle LA, Rainey BJ, et al. Single nucleotide polymorphisms in the methylenetetrahydrofolate reductase gene are common in US Caucasian and Hispanic American populations. Int J Mol Med 2001;8(5):509–11.
29. Krabbendam I, Dekker GA. Pregnancy outcome in patients with a history of recurrent spontaneous miscarriages and documented thrombophilias. Gynecol Obstet Invest 2004;57(3):127–31.
30. den Heijer M, Rosendaal FR, Blom HJ, et al. Hyperhomocysteinemia and venous thrombosis: a meta-analysis. Thromb Haemost 1998;80(6):874–7.
31. Eichinger S. Homocysteine, vitamin B6 and the risk of recurrent venous thromboembolism. Pathophysiol Haemost Thromb 2003;33(5–6):342–4.
32. den Heijer M, Willems HP, Blom HJ, et al. Homocysteine lowering by B vitamins and the secondary prevention of deep vein thrombosis and pulmonary embolism: a randomized, placebo-controlled, double-blind trial. Blood 2007;109(1):139–44.
33. Bezemer ID, Doggen CJ, Vos HL, et al. No association between the common MTHFR 677C->T polymorphism and venous thrombosis: results from the MEGA study. Arch Intern Med 2007;167(5):497–501.
34. Nurk E, Tell GS, Refsum H, et al. Associations between maternal methylenetetrahydrofolate reductase polymorphisms and adverse outcomes of pregnancy: the Hordaland Homocysteine Study. Am J Med 2004;117(1):26–31.

35. Molloy AM, Mills JL, Kirke PN, et al. Folate status and neural tube defects. Biofactors 1999;10(2–3):291–4.
36. Ceyhan ST, Beyan C, Bahce M, et al. Thrombophilia-associated gene mutations in women with pregnancies complicated by fetal neural tube defects. Int J Gynaecol Obstet 2008;101(2):188–9.
37. Akar N, Akar E, Deda G, et al. Spina bifida and common mutations at the homocysteine metabolism pathway. Clin Genet 2000;57(3):230–1.
38. Molloy AM, Weir DG, Scott JM. Homocysteine, folate enzymes and neural tube defects. Haematologica 1999;84(Suppl EHA-4):53–6.
39. Coulam CB, Jeyendran RS, Fishel LA, et al. Multiple thrombophilic gene mutations rather than specific gene mutations are risk factors for recurrent miscarriage. Am J Reprod Immunol 2006;55(5):360–8.
40. Kutteh WH, Triplett DA. Thrombophilias and recurrent pregnancy loss. Semin Reprod Med 2006;24(1):54–66.
41. Brenner B, Sarig G, Weiner Z, et al. Thrombophilic polymorphisms are common in women with fetal loss without apparent cause. Thromb Haemost 1999;82(1):6–9.
42. Sarig G, Younis JS, Hoffman R, et al. Thrombophilia is common in women with idiopathic pregnancy loss and is associated with late pregnancy wastage. Fertil Steril 2002;77(2):342–7.
43. Kupferminc MJ, Eldor A, Steinman N, et al. Increased frequency of genetic thrombophilia in women with complications of pregnancy. N Engl J Med 1999;340(1):9–13.
44. Castoldi E, Simioni P, Kalafatis M, et al. Combinations of 4 mutations (FV R506Q, FV H1299R, FV Y1702C, PT 20210G/A) affecting the prothrombinase complex in a thrombophilic family. Blood 2000;96(4):1443–8.
45. Infante-Rivard C, David M, Gauthier R, et al. Lupus anticoagulants, anticardiolipin antibodies, and fetal loss. A case-control study. N Engl J Med 1991;325(15):1063–6.
46. Lockshin MD. Pregnancy loss in the antiphospholipid syndrome. Thromb Haemost 1999;82(2):641–8.
47. James A. Practice bulletin no. 123: thromboembolism in pregnancy. Obstet Gynecol 2011;118(3):718–29.
48. Lonn E, Yusuf S, Arnold MJ, et al. Homocysteine lowering with folic acid and B vitamins in vascular disease. N Engl J Med 2006;354(15):1567–77.

Recurrent Miscarriage Clinics

M.M.J. Van den Berg, MD, Rosa Vissenberg, MD,
Mariëtte Goddijn, MD, PhD*

KEYWORDS

- Recurrent miscarriage • Recurrent miscarriage clinic • Quality of care
- Guideline adherence • Patient preferences

KEY POINTS

- A recurrent miscarriage (RM) clinic offers specialist investigation and treatment of women with recurrent first- and second-trimester miscarriage.
- RM care preferably should be provided by only one doctor per couple.
- A treatment strategy should be designed with the couple for a subsequent pregnancy.
- Evidence-based guidelines are necessary for the facilitation of evidence-based practice and to reduce practice variation between professionals.
- Guideline adherence can be achieved by implementation efforts.

INTRODUCTION

A miscarriage is the spontaneous loss of a clinically established intrauterine pregnancy before the fetus has reached viability. It includes pregnancy losses until the maximum of 24 weeks of gestation.[1] Between 10% and 15% of all clinically recognized pregnancies result in a spontaneous miscarriage. However, the overall prevalence of pregnancy losses, including biochemical pregnancies, is generally assumed 4 to 5 times higher.[1] Approximately one-quarter of all women experience at least one miscarriage during their lives.[2,3] In conclusion, a miscarriage is a frequent event and it is known that a miscarriage has a huge impact on a patient's life.

Up to 5% of all couples face recurrent miscarriage (RM). The definition may vary but starts when at least two or more miscarriages have occurred.[4,5] The sequence of the miscarriages is not necessarily consecutive.[4,6]

A RM clinic offers specialist investigation and treatment of women with recurrent first- and second-trimester miscarriages. It is an outpatient clinic with reproductive

The authors have nothing to disclose.
Department of Obstetrics and Gynecology, Center for Reproductive Medicine, Academic Medical Center, H4-205, PO Box 22660, Amsterdam 1100 DD, The Netherlands
* Corresponding author.
E-mail address: m.goddijn@amc.nl

gynecologists specialized in evidence-based RM care. This consultant-led clinic provides a dedicated and focused service to couples who have experienced at least two prior miscarriages.

GUIDELINES
Guideline Adherence

To improve the quality of care for RM, guidelines have been developed. These guidelines address the facilitation of evidence-based practice and reduce practice variation between professionals.[7] Couples with RM are often not treated according to the most up-to-date clinical evidence, as summarized in recent guidelines.[8,9] Ineffective management of couples with RM is caused by underdiagnostics as well as overdiagnostics, resulting in unnecessary tests and costs.[10] This barrier and other barriers to RM management are shown in **Box 1**. The introduction of new guidelines alone is not enough to prevent this ineffective management. Guideline implementation research shows that to achieve a high level of guideline adherence, implementation efforts are necessary.[11,12] So far, it is not obvious which implementation strategy to apply to improve guideline adherence and, meanwhile, quality of care in couples with RM.

Guideline adherence could be improved with a multifaceted implementation strategy. In total, 23 quality indicators for care in couples with RM have been identified.[13] These can be used to measure and monitor care for RM patients. These guidelines improved remarkably after introduction of the developed implementation strategy.[13]

Another essential step in the implementation process of guidelines is qualitative research to identify barriers to and facilitators for guideline adherence.[7,11] One study identified barriers in management of RM in four domains: the guidelines, professionals, patients, and organization by semistructured interview among professionals and patients.[14] The most important identified barriers for guideline adherence were the guidelines being too complicated, lack of up-to-date patient information, and lack of detailed knowledge about family history.[14] Based on the detected

---

Box 1
Barriers to high-quality RM management

Guidelines

- The definition of RM differs: two versus three miscarriages and consecutive versus non-consecutive miscarriage.
- Few good RCTs have been performed to investigate diagnostic and treatment options.

Organization

- Not every hospital has a recurrent miscarriage clinic/early pregnancy unit.
- Not every hospital works with a RM expert.
- Not every hospital offers participation in RCTs.

Professionals

- Doctors want to offer treatment despite a lack of evidence.

Patients

- Patients have a strong will to perform diagnostic tests despite a lack of evidence.
- Patients have a strong will to start treatment despite a lack of evidence.

determinants for nonadherence and the barriers experienced by professionals and patients, an implementation strategy for improvement could be developed.

Guidelines state that all couples who suffer from RM should be offered advice and referred to a specialist clinic with appropriately trained health care professionals.[15] Couples with unexplained RM should be informed about their individual chances of success in a next pregnancy.[16] Tender loving care (TLC) and health advice are the two established treatments of RM (discussed later).[7] Health advice includes intake of folic acid, restriction of the intake of coffee, stopping smoking and drinking alcohol, and lifestyle advice and/or dietary measures in cases of overweight.[7] For women with RM and a subsequent confirmed pregnancy test, arrangements should be in place for an ultrasound scan and for receiving shared antenatal care in a high-risk obstetric clinic.[15] It is extremely important that all staff dealing with RM couples are trained in emotional aspects of pregnancy loss. In this way, immediate support can be provided and patients have direct access to specialist counseling.[15] The aim is to make all health professionals providing early pregnancy care aware of the current approach to this problem.[17]

LOGISTICAL REQUIREMENTS

Couples who have suffered two or more miscarriages should be referred to a RM clinic. **Fig. 1** provides a flowchart for the entry in a RM clinic. Preferably a patient information brochure has been sent to couples before their first visit to the clinic. This way, a couple's expectations can be met. **Box 2** and **Fig. 2** give an overview of the tools provided by RM clinics.

Location

The service is often situated in a gynecology outpatient clinic or near an early pregnancy unit. Avoid, whenever possible, locating a clinic near an antenatal clinic to reduce any distress experienced by women seeing ongoing pregnancies while waiting.

Rooms

A room is necessary for taking history and examination. It is important that the room can be locked to guarantee privacy while women are changing and being examined. In certain units, a separate room is used to perform the transvaginal sonography. These rooms should be warm and have good lighting for vaginal examinations. Another separate room for breaking bad news may be valuable. In this way, women are allowed to have some time to reflect and compose themselves before proceeding with further management. It is preferable that this room has telephone access to allow calls to relatives or friends.

Staffing

All RM clinics should have a consultant with a special interest in RM. RM care should be provided by only one doctor per couple. Multidisciplinary support should be provided by other departments, such as clinical genetics, an early pregnancy assessment unit, pathology, radiology, internal medicine, endocrinology, and/or hematology departments. It is important that all staff dealing with RM couples are trained in emotional aspects of pregnancy loss. In this way, immediate support can be provided and every couple has direct access to specialist counseling.[15] The aim is to make all health professionals providing early pregnancy care aware of the current approach to manage RM.[17]

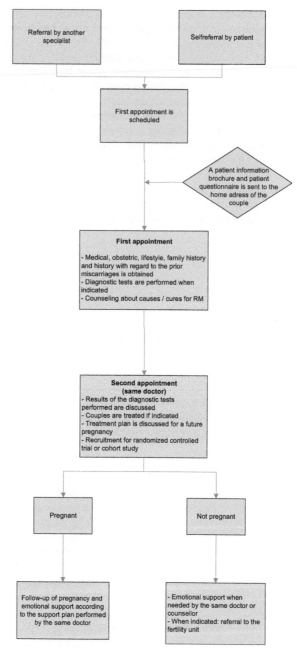

Fig. 1. Flowchart for entry into an RM clinic.

Equipment

For follow-up of a future pregnancy to confirm a miscarriage, the ability to perform transvaginal and/or transabdominal scan is necessary. It is preferable that the ultrasound has the ability to store copies of all images to be given to the women if

---

Box 2
Tools for recurrent miscarriage clinics

- A RM specific protocol for diagnosis & treatment should be available so that all couples receive the same standard care that is in line with the information on the patient information brochure.
- Proper work-up for diagnosis and treatment is indicated.
- Unproven therapies should be used only in the setting of a properly conducted randomized trial.
- Couples with unexplained RM should be informed about their individual chances of success in a next pregnancy.
- A plan should be made how to offer good support during the first trimester in the next pregnancy.
- Because the chance of a successful pregnancy is still promising, treatment should focus on supportive care, where possible.
- Involve the male partner.
- Couple-based psychological care should be offered to couples with RM.
- An RM clinic should preferably be organized in a way that couples receive individual care from one doctor per couple.
- A patient information brochure must be available and preferably sent to couples before their first visit, so they know what to expect from the RM clinic.

---

requested. Also an electronic database is advisable for documentation of all images. This gives an opportunity to exchange images with an early pregnancy unit.

Record Keeping

History, examination, and scan findings need to be documented and archived in the women's patient notes or in a database that is secured with a password-based access. A standardized protocol should be used for the documentation of history and examination. This way, all patients are asked the same questions and the chance of forgetting something is low.

Laboratory Services

A basic requirement is access to hematology and biochemistry to facilitate RM diagnostic work-up.

One-Stop Recurrent Miscarriage Clinics

Some clinics are organized as an one-stop RM clinic.[18] When a couple is referred to a RM clinic, they receive a letter with a set of investigation forms and are advised to take blood tests. This way, the results of the blood tests are known and can be discussed when the couple attends the clinic for the first time. During the same consultation, history and physical examination are documented, which leads to a management plan. Couples only attend the RM clinic once and do not need any unnecessary repeat consultations. Before leaving the clinic, each couple is seen by a nurse counselor. They are given a direct telephone number to the antenatal assessment area (AAA), where all pregnancies are followed-up by the counselor. When a couple is pregnant, they call the AAA to receive follow-up scans and antenatal care. This one-stop clinic reduced the interval of visits by 36% (206.6–130.4 days; $P<.001$) and reduced the number of visits by 60% (2.5–1; $P<.002$).[18] This approach

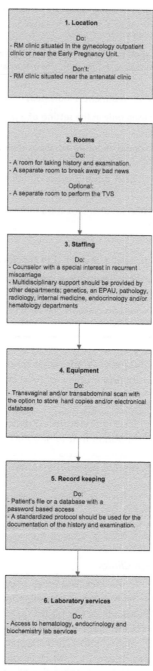

Fig. 2. Flowchart of logistical requirements for a RM clinic.

provides no patient-centered care, however. There is no explanation as to which diagnostic test is performed. Also, not all couples need to go through all diagnostic tests. Preferably, diagnostic work-up is based on proper history taking and individually tailored. Most diagnostic tests should only be performed on indication.

DOCTOR PREFERENCES
Diagnostic Tests

When a couple is seen at first consultation for RM, a detailed history is taken with regard to prior miscarriages and medical, obstetric, lifestyle, and family history. The decision to perform diagnostic investigations depends on the medical history. Diagnostic tests should only be carried out if the test can either give insight in the prognosis of an individual patient or if the established cause can be treated effectively. Diagnostic tests are performed and treatments are described despite a lack of evidence. Before introducing new diagnostic investigations in clinical practice, these tests should be evaluated thoroughly. The increasing costs of health care have been calling for elimination of ineffective medical testing.[10] Women with RM are often desperate and can be demanding. In clinical practice, it has been shown that too many diagnostic investigations and unproved treatments are performed in women with RM. This is a result of doctors who find it difficult to resist insistent women.[8]

Many of the diagnostic tests available for couples with RM give no information with regard to the prognosis in a future pregnancy. There is also a lack of evidence of potential treatment options in cases of a positive test result. Therefore, there is a need for evidenced-based guidelines, based on prospective cohort studies for prognostic purposes and randomized controlled trials (RCTs) to investigate the usefulness of the treatment options available for RM couples.

Work-Up

The guidelines of the Association of Early Pregnancy Units suggest that patients should not be subjected to tests without a proper plan of further follow-up and management (www.earlypregnancy.org.uk). It is important that both partners are aware of what is going to happen. The couple should be prepared for the fact that in a majority of cases no cause is found for the RM. Encourage the partner's participation and encourage the couple to talk about their fears and anxieties. Diagnostic testing should not be done only to reassure patients that something is being done. If diagnostic tests are performed, make sure that an explanation is given of all tests before taking blood samples. Reassure the couple that all known risk factors for RM will be explored. Discuss lifestyle end preconceptual care with the couple as available treatment plans. This prepares the couple for their future consultation. If a couple achieves a pregnancy, a doctor should arrange ultrasound scanning at 6 weeks' gestation and thereafter every week or 2 weeks, after discussing with the couple, for maternal assurance until seen in the antenatal booking clinic (www.earlypregnancy.org.uk). It is important to discuss a treatment plan for a future pregnancy with the couple. Not all couples want to have an ultrasound scan every other week. It is important that the doctor listens to the patient.[19,20] Management of women with RM based on emotional support supplemurrent approach to this proented by ultrasound scan in early pregnancy has success rates of between 70% and 80%. Individual changes depend on the number of prior miscarriages and, more importantly, female age.[21,22]

Scientific Research Programs

For more than 50% of women with RM, no underlying cause is found. This is frustrating for couples but also for clinicians and, therefore, it is tempting to start empiric treatment. Treatments of the RM population are often introduced without evaluating effectiveness. The only way to improve quality of care, however, is to apply an evidence-based approach.

Scientific research is necessary to study the effectiveness of new interventions, to study patient preferences, and to evaluate health care and costs or other outcomes. Cooperation between multiple centers, nationally and internationally, will facilitate research projects. Research networks will improve the infrastructure for scientific studies. This leads to a faster recruitment of patients in trials and better and faster implementation of study results but also standardization of care.

Patient data of women visiting the RM clinics should be recorded in databases to obtain large cohorts of RM patients. These anonymous data can be used for both scientific research projects and evaluation of health care.

PATIENT PREFERENCES
Psychological and Relational Consequences of Recurrent Miscarriage

Experiencing RM can be a traumatic event and is often accompanied by negative emotional distress.[23] Different psychological and psychiatric effects can be induced. Feelings of grief, lowered self-esteem, guilt, anger, and depression and anxiety disorders are common after miscarriage but also during the subsequent pregnancy.[24,25] Anxiety is the predominant response to RM.[25–27] Different prevalence rates have been described for depressive symptoms, varying from 10% to 30%.[27–30] Symptoms of anxiety and depression can be present for 6 months after a pregnancy loss.[25,28,31]

Psychological reactions and grief reactions after RM are different in women than in men. Women are more distressed than men after RM and men have lower anxiety levels.[24,32,33] Unlike women, men do not react with an increased depressive reaction. Men grieve but less intensely and enduringly than their partners.[24] Some men feel burdened by their wives' grief or depressive reactions.[31] These gender differences may worsen or have a negative impact on the psychological adjustment and marital relationships in RM couples. Conflicting reactions may affect couples' interactions and promote depressive reactions in the women. Low marital adjustment and sexual changes after RM have been reported.[24,27] Data on whether a couple's relationship is adversely affected by RM are conflicting. One study does not describe a negative impact on the relationship.[24] But there is also evidence that women with a history of RM were at a higher risk of their relationships ending compared with women without a history of miscarriage.[34]

Supportive Care

A majority of women with RM are classified as having unexplained RM. For these patients, no effective treatment intervention exists. Current guidelines advise supportive care for women with (unexplained) RM during the next pregnancy.[7] The guidelines of the Association of Early Pregnancy Units suggest that all staff members should be trained in emotional aspects of early pregnancy loss and offer bereavement counseling (www.earlypregnancy.org.uk). Offering so-called TLC, which consists of reassurance and psychological support, has led to an improvement in pregnancy outcome after unexplained RM in controlled studies.[16,21,22,35] Live birth rates up to 85% have been reported after supportive care. These studies were of low quality, however, because a clear definition of TLC is lacking and the study populations were too small. The supportive care offered in earlier studies varied widely and no clear definition of supportive care exists. How supportive care is defined and experienced depends on the perception of clinicians and patients and, therefore, is difficult to analyze as a clear outcome measure.

Because pregnancy-related fear may have a negative impact on the course of pregnancy and delivery, interventions to reduce anxiety are highly recommended.[36] It is not clear from the literature whether anxiety might be reduced due to supportive care or treatment in an RM clinic. One study showed that offering supportive care in a RM clinic does not significantly change anxiety levels.[26] This was only investigated in one study and the study population was too small to draw final conclusions about reduction of anxiety levels by supportive care.

There is limited evidence on the effect of RM clinics on psychological outcomes. Possible explanations for this are that supportive care should be more accurately defined and that analyzing supportive care as an outcome remains difficult.

Patient Preferences and Perspectives

Women's perceptions and preferences for supportive care options have been studied in qualitative and quantitative research.[19,20] Women with RM prefer the following supportive care option for their next pregnancy: a plan with one doctor, who shows understanding, takes them seriously, has knowledge of their obstetric history, listens to them, gives information about RM, shows empathy, informs on progress, and enquires about emotional needs. Also, there is a need for ultrasound examination during symptoms, directly after a positive pregnancy test, and every 2 weeks. If a miscarriage occurs, most women prefer to talk to a medical or psychological professional afterward. A majority of women have a low preference for admission to a hospital.[20]

Couples do not always experience the supportive care of health professionals as optimal.[31] An important task for clinicians is to discuss with couples what their preferences are for supportive care and to make a plan for the next pregnancy. This improves patient-centered care.

RECOMMENDATIONS

RM patients are vulnerable and should receive good clinical supportive care. A RM clinic is necessary to provide this care. Couples can be guided by one doctor and a plan can be made together with the couples for a future pregnancy. Also, by working with a specific protocol, all patients receive the same standard care.

All women who present with RM should have access to a specialized RM clinic with appropriately trained health care professionals.[15]

REFERENCES

1. Rai R, Regan L. Recurrent miscarriage. Lancet 2006;368(9535):601–11.
2. Stephenson M, Kutteh W. Evaluation and management of recurrent early pregnancy loss. Clin Obstet Gynecol 2007;50(1):132–45.
3. Stern JJ, Dorfmann AD, Gutierrez-Najar AJ, et al. Frequency of abnomral karyotypes among abortuses from women with and withouw a history of recurrent spontaneous abortion. Fertil Steril 1996;65(2):250–3.
4. Jaslow CR, Carney JL, Kutteh WH. Diagnostic factors identified in 1020 women with two versus three or more recurrent pregnancy losses. Fertil Steril 2010; 93(4):1234–43.
5. Raijcan-Separovic E, Qiao Y, Tyson C, et al. Genomic changes detected by array CGH in human embryos with developmental defects. Mol Hum Reprod 2010; 16(2):125–34.
6. van den Boogaard E, Kaandorp SP, Franssen MT, et al. Consecutive or nonconsecutive recurrent miscarriage: is there any difference in carrier status? Humanit Rep 2010;25(6):1411–4.

7. Jauniaux E, Farquharson RG, Christiansen OB, et al. Evidence-based guidelines for the investigation and medical treatment of recurrent miscarriage. Hum Reprod 2006;21(9):2216–22.

8. Franssen MT, Korevaar JC, van der Veen F, et al. Management of recurrent miscarriage: evaluating the impact of a guideline. Hum Reprod 2007;22(5): 1298–303.

9. van den Boogaard E, Hermens RP, Verhoeve HR, et al. Selective karyotyping in recurrent miscarriage: are recommended guidelines adopted in daily clinical practice? Hum Reprod 2011;26(8):1965–70.

10. Berwick DM, Hackbarth AD. Eliminating waste in US health care. JAMA 2012; 307(14):1513–6.

11. Bero LA, Grilli R, Grimshaw JM, et al. Closing the gap between research and practice: an overview of systematic reviews of interventions to promote the implementation of research findings. The Cochrane Effective Practice and Organization of Care Review Group. BMJ 1998;317(7156):465–8.

12. Grol R. Personal paper. Beliefs and evidence in changing clinical practice. BMJ 1997;315(7105):418–21.

13. van den Boogaard E, Goddijn M, Leschot NJ, et al. Development of guideline-based quality indicators for recurrent miscarriage. Reprod Biomed Online 2010;20(2):267–73.

14. van den Boogaard E, Hermens RP, Leschot NJ, et al. Identification of barriers for good adherence to a guideline on recurrent miscarriage. Acta Obstet Gynecol Scand 2011;90(2):186–91.

15. Royal college of obstetricians and gynaecologists. Standards for gynaeacology: chapter 4 recurrent miscarriage. 2008. Available at: http://www.rcog.org.uk/womens-health/clinical-guidance/investigation-and-treatment-couples-recurrent-miscarriage-green-top-.

16. Brigham SA, Conlon C, Farquharson RG. A longitudinal study of pregnancy outcome following idiopathic recurrent miscarriage. Hum Reprod 1999;14(11):2868–71.

17. Guidelines on the management of women with recurrent miscarriage. Association of early pregnancy units. 2007. Available at: http://www.ptmp.pl/archives/apm/13-4/APM134-guidelines-7-28.pdf.

18. Habayeb OM, Konje JC. The one-stop recurrent miscarriage clinic: an evaluation of its effectiveness and outcome. Hum Reprod 2004;19(12):2952–8.

19. Musters AM, Taminiau-Bloem EF, van den Boogaard E, et al. Supportive care for women with unexplained recurrent miscarriage: patients' perspectives. Hum Reprod 2011;26(4):873–7.

20. Musters AM, Koot YE, van den Boogaard NM, et al. Supportive care for women with recurrent miscarriage: a survey to quantify women's preferences. Hum Reprod 2013;28(2):398–405.

21. Clifford K, Rai R, Regan L. Future pregnancy outcome in unexplained recurrent first trimester miscarriage. Hum Reprod 1997;12(2):387–9.

22. Liddell HS, Pattison NS, Zanderigo A. Recurrent miscarriage–outcome after supportive care in early pregnancy. Aust N Z J Obstet Gynaecol 1991;31(4):320–2.

23. Lee C, Slade P. Miscarriage as a traumatic event: a review of the literature and new implications for intervention. J Psychosom Res 1996;40(3):235–44.

24. Serrano F, Lima ML. Recurrent miscarriage: psychological and relational consequences for couples. Psychol Psychother 2006;79(Pt 4):585–94.

25. Geller PA, Kerns D, Klier CM. Anxiety following miscarriage and the subsequent pregnancy: a review of the literature and future directions. J Psychosom Res 2004;56(1):35–45.

26. Mevorach-Zussman N, Bolotin A, Shalev H, et al. Anxiety and deterioration of quality of life factors associated with recurrent miscarriage in an observational study. J Perinat Med 2012;40(5):495–501.
27. Klock SC, Chang G, Hiley A, et al. Psychological distress among women with recurrent spontaneous abortion. Psychosomatics 1997;38(5):503–7.
28. Neugebauer R, Kline J, Shrout P, et al. Major depressive disorder in the 6 months after miscarriage. JAMA 1997;277(5):383–8.
29. Craig M, Tata P, Regan L. Psychiatric morbidity among patients with recurrent miscarriage. J Psychosom Obstet Gynaecol 2002;23(3):157–64.
30. Thapar AK, Thapar A. Psychological sequelae of miscarriage: a controlled study using the general health questionnaire and the hospital anxiety and depression scale. Br J Gen Pract 1992;42(356):94–6.
31. Conway K, Russell G. Couples' grief and experience of support in the aftermath of miscarriage. Br J Med Psychol 2000;73(Pt 4):531–45.
32. Beutel M, Willner H, Deckardt R, et al. Similarities and differences in couples' grief reactions following a miscarriage: results from a longitudinal study. J Psychosom Res 1996;40(3):245–53.
33. Kagami M, Maruyama T, Koizumi T, et al. Psychological adjustment and psychosocial stress among Japanese couples with a history of recurrent pregnancy loss. Hum Reprod 2012;27(3):787–94.
34. Sugiura-Ogasawara M, Suzuki S, Ozaki Y, et al. Frequency of recurrent spontaneous abortion and its influence on further marital relationship and illness: the Okazaki Cohort Study in Japan. J Obstet Gynaecol Res 2013;39(1):126–31.
35. Stray-Pedersen B, Stray-Pedersen S. Etiologic factors and subsequent reproductive performance in 195 couples with a prior history of habitual abortion. Am J Obstet Gynecol 1984;148(2):140–6.
36. Fertl KI, Bergner A, Beyer R, et al. Levels and effects of different forms of anxiety during pregnancy after a prior miscarriage. Eur J Obstet Gynecol Reprod Biol 2009;142(1):23–9.

Unexplained Recurrent Pregnancy Loss

Sotirios H. Saravelos, MBBS, Lesley Regan, MBBS, MD, FRCOG*

KEYWORDS

- Idiopathic • Miscarriage • Pregnancy loss • Recurrent • Unexplained

KEY POINTS

- Women with unexplained recurrent pregnancy loss (RPL) represent a highly heterogeneous group of patients.
- Some women will have suffered RPL attributable to chance alone, and will therefore have a good future prognosis, whereas others will have a genuine pathologic condition that cannot be identified by the current investigative protocols, and will have a comparatively worse prognosis.
- The definition used to diagnose RPL, specifically the number and type of previous miscarriages and maternal age, will significantly affect not only the incidence of women with RPL but also the proportion of women with unexplained RPL.
- Past studies have investigated systemic endocrine and immunologic mechanisms as potential causes for pregnancy loss in unexplained RPL, while exciting new work has focused on spermatozoal, embryonic, and endometrial characteristics to explain the regulation of implantation and subsequent pregnancy loss.
- In the clinical and research context, stratification of women with unexplained RPL according to whether they have a high probability of pathologic status will help select women who are most appropriate for further investigation and potential future treatment.

THE IMPORTANCE OF THE DEFINITION

Recurrent pregnancy loss (RPL) is a heterogeneous condition that encompasses a mixed cohort of women with different reproductive histories and a large range of conditions.[1] Unlike other diagnoses, the definition and diagnosis of RPL is a rather arbitrary one, which is often the reason why different clinicians or bodies may use different and interchangeable terms to characterize women with pregnancy losses, for example:

Sporadic pregnancy loss (SPL): 1 miscarriage <24 weeks
Recurrent early pregnancy loss (REPL): 2 or more miscarriages <10 weeks

The authors have no conflicts of interest with regard to this work.
Department of Obstetrics and Gynaecology, St Mary's Campus, Imperial College London, Mint Wing, South Wharf Road, London W2 1PG, UK
* Corresponding author.
E-mail address: l.regan@imperial.ac.uk

Obstet Gynecol Clin N Am 41 (2014) 157–166
http://dx.doi.org/10.1016/j.ogc.2013.10.008
obgyn.theclinics.com

Recurrent pregnancy loss (RPL): 2 or more miscarriages <24 weeks
Recurrent early miscarriage (REM): 3 or more consecutive miscarriages <10 weeks
Recurrent miscarriage (RM): 3 or more consecutive miscarriages <24 weeks

The main differences observed in varying terminologies used are (1) the number of miscarriages and (2) the types of miscarriages (ie, early vs late). In the context of both research and clinical practice, the number and types of miscarriages that are used in a definition are extremely important, as they may result in different cohorts of patients with different abnormalities, different prognoses, and different health care needs. As a result, the definition used to diagnose RPL has a direct effect on the profile of women who will eventually have a diagnosis of unexplained RPL.

Number of Miscarriages Suffered

If we accept that the average rate of sporadic miscarriage is approximately 15% in the general population,[2] then depending on the number of miscarriages that are required to make the diagnosis of RPL, the theoretical incidence of the condition changes (**Table 1**). For example, if 2 miscarriages are used for the definition of RPL, 2% (0.15^2) or more of women will have the condition, whereas if 5 or more miscarriages are used for the definition, as little as 0.01% (0.15^5) of women may have the condition. Traditionally, the American Society for Reproductive Medicine (ASRM) has accepted 2 or more pregnancy losses as part of the definition,[3] whereas the European Society for Human Reproduction and Embryology (ESHRE) has used 3 or more pregnancy losses in their definition.[4] For the purpose of this article, both 2 and 3 miscarriages are discussed as part of the definition.

Types of Miscarriages Suffered

Another important element of the definition, which again would affect both the incidence and profile of patients diagnosed with RPL, is the type of pregnancy losses included in the definition of RPL. The most important question is whether biochemical pregnancy losses should be considered as part of the definition for RPL. Most bodies make clear that only clinical pregnancies should be part of the definition, and the ASRM is a good example because it states that pregnancy losses should include only those that can be documented by ultrasonographic or histopathologic

Table 1
Theoretical incidence of recurrent pregnancy loss (RPL) according to the number of miscarriages used in the definition

No. of Miscarriages Required to Diagnose RPL	Incidence ≥
2	1/45
3	1/300
4	1/2000
5	1/13,000
6	1/90,000
7	1/600,000
8	1/4,000,000

Estimates based on a mean sporadic miscarriage rate of 15%.
Incidences calculated as $I = \mu^{number\ of\ miscarriages}$ (where μ = sporadic miscarriage rate of 15%).
Incidences may be underestimated, as the true incidence of RPL is thought to be more than the theoretical incidence.

examination.[3] The reason for this is that biochemical pregnancy losses have been shown to be very common in the general population, with almost 60% to 80% of pregnancies thought to end in an early preclinical loss.[5,6] Despite this, clinicians may still find it difficult to exclude these pregnancies from the definition of RPL, particularly if women have used sensitive over-the-counter tests to identify early pregnancies and are subsequently anxious for investigations following repeated biochemical losses.

However, if put into context, it can be estimated that almost 20% (0.6^3) of women in the general population may experience 3 biochemical pregnancy losses attributable to chance alone,[7] most of which will not need investigating.

Maternal Age

Most definitions of RPL will not include the age of the woman. However, maternal age is perhaps the single most important determinant of miscarriage in the general and the RPL populations,[2,8] which is invariably a result of oocyte and embryonic aneuploidy.[9] As a result, the age of the women will affect the incidence of the condition (**Table 2**). For example, the theoretical incidence of RPL (2 pregnancy losses) in women younger than 25 years is approximately 1.2% (SPL rate of 0.11^2), whereas for women of 45 years or older it may exceed 50% (SPL rate of 0.75^2).

INCIDENCE
Unexplained Recurrent Pregnancy Loss

Although the exact incidence of RPL has never been reliably determined, most investigators would agree that the overall incidence of RPL (2 or more pregnancy losses) is approximately 3%, whereas that of RM (3 or more miscarriages) is approximately 1% of the population.[10] From these data, it is deduced that approximately 50% of women will suffer from unexplained RPL.[11,12] However, just as the factors mentioned previously (ie, number of miscarriages, types of miscarriages, and maternal age) will affect the incidence of RPL, they will also affect the proportion of women that will be diagnosed with unexplained RPL. For example, if women older than 40 years are selected, not only will there be a higher incidence of women diagnosed with RPL (at least 25%), but the majority, approximately 65%, will have suffered miscarriages resulting from embryonic chromosomal anomalies, most commonly aneuploidy,[13] and therefore very few may be truly unexplained. In fact, they will be healthy women with recurrent SPL with no additional abnormality or, otherwise, women with RPL attributable to chance alone. Paradoxically, if there are no cytogenetics available when the patient

Table 2	
Theoretical incidence of RPL (2 pregnancy losses) according to maternal age	
Maternal Age	**Incidence of RPL ≥**
20	1/85
25	1/70
30	1/45
35	1/16
40	1/4
45	1/2

Estimates based on a sporadic miscarriage rates according to maternal age.
Incidences calculated as $I = \mu^2$ (where μ = sporadic miscarriage rates for age).
Incidences may be underestimated, as the true incidence of RPL is thought to be more than the theoretical incidence.

presents to the clinic (which often is the case), most will be diagnosed as having unexplained RPL, as these patients are unlikely to have any abnormalities identified on routine testing. This situation shows the importance of distinguishing between healthy women with RPL attributable to chance alone (secondary to aneuploidy) and women with genuine unexplained RPL that may have a treatable disorder other than aneuploidy.

Recurrent Pregnancy Loss Attributable to Chance

In any cohort of women with RPL, a proportion of women will have suffered sporadic RPL that can be attributed to chance alone.[7,14] As mentioned previously, these women will not have any additional abnormality, their routine investigations will be negative, and they will invariably be diagnosed as having unexplained RPL. It is therefore very important to distinguish between women with sporadic RPL attributable to chance and women with genuine unexplained RPL as it may be only the latter that require investigation and treatment.

To estimate the proportion of women with RPL who have suffered from RPL that is due to chance alone, the incidence of SPL in the general population needs to be identified[2] followed by the rates of recurrent SPL (occurring from chance alone) using the assumption that if SPL rate = μ, recurrent SPL rate = μ^n, where n = number of miscarriages (**Table 3**). When performing this analysis for women aged 30 to 35 years, it is shown that 2.25% will have suffered 2 SPL resulting from chance, whereas 0.34% will have suffered 3 SPL attributable to chance alone. Given that the total incidence of RPL and RM is thought to be 1% and 3%, respectively, it can be assumed that up to 75% (2.25/3) of women with RPL may have suffered 2 RPL attributable to chance alone, whereas up to 35% (0.34/1) may have suffered 3 RPL that is due to chance alone.

THE CAUSES OF UNEXPLAINED RECURRENT PREGNANCY LOSS
The Factor of Chance

As already mentioned, a significant number of women will have suffered RPL because of chance alone and will not have any identifiable abnormality other than embryonic aneuploidy, which may not have been tested before the referral to a specialist clinic. These patients are healthy women who have been unlucky in their pursuit of a pregnancy, and will be diagnosed as having unexplained RPL because their investigations will be invariably normal. These women are also those with a very good prognosis in their future pregnancy without the need for surgical or pharmacologic intervention.

Table 3
Incidence of RPL occurring by chance for women with 1, 2, and 3 miscarriages

Age (y)	Recurrent Pregnancy Loss Rates (Occurring by Chance) (%)		
	1 Miscarriage	2 Miscarriages	3 Miscarriages
20–24	11	1.21	0.13
25–29	12	1.44	0.17
30–34	15	2.25	0.34
35–39	25	6.25	1.56

Data from Saravelos SH, Li TC. Unexplained recurrent miscarriage: how can we explain it? Hum Rep 2012;27(7):1882–6; and Nybo Andersen AM, Wohlfahrt J, Christens P, et al. Maternal age and fetal loss: population-based register linkage study. BMJ 2000;320(7251):1708–12.

This proposition is supported by well-conducted randomized controlled trials (RCTs) and meta-analyses, which have shown that treatment such as aspirin, heparin, and intravenous immunoglobulin does not improve pregnancy outcomes in women with unexplained RPL.[15,16]

Of course, not all women with unexplained RPL will have suffered their pregnancy losses attributable to chance alone, and a certain proportion will have pathologic conditions other than embryonic aneuploidy that will not be detected by the current investigation protocols. These women, typically younger, will go on to suffer higher order of miscarriages (4, 5, or more) and are the most challenging to manage.

The Egg

Although it is accepted that aneuploidy is the main cause for pregnancy loss in women with increased maternal age, it has been speculated that some women with unexplained RPL may suffer from premature ovarian aging, leading to reduced oocyte quality and quantity. Although oocyte quantity and quality cannot be easily assessed, one group compared basal follicle-stimulating hormone (FSH) in women with unexplained RPL and in controls as an indirect means of assessing for premature ovarian aging and decline in oocyte quality.[17] Their results showed comparable basal FSH levels for both groups across all ages up to 40 years.

Another group reported on oocyte donations of 8 couples with unexplained RPL who had poor response to ovarian hyperstimulation.[18] This study is interesting, as oocyte donation could theoretically reduce the risk of pregnancy loss in women suffering from RPL attributable to oocyte and embryonic aneuploidy. The investigators reported a rate of 11.1% pregnancy loss in these 8 cycles, and questioned whether the oocyte, rather than maternal and paternal factors, is the origin of RPL. Unfortunately, although these preliminary findings are exciting, there is an urgent need for further controlled follow-up studies.

The Sperm

The role of the sperm in unexplained RPL remains controversial, with varying original reports on factors such as Y-chromosome microdeletions, sperm oxidative stress, sperm DNA fragmentation, sperm concentration, morphology, and function.[19] More recently, a systematic review and meta-analysis reported that DNA fragmentation was indeed significantly associated with miscarriage, and concluded that using methods to select sperm without DNA damage may reduce miscarriage in assisted conception treatment.[20] The implications of these findings for the unexplained RPL population are still open to debate.

The Embryo

Similar to reducing the risk of chromosomal abnormalities by focusing on the egg and sperm, it has been thought that artificial reproductive technology (ART), and specifically preimplantation genetic screening (PGS) of the embryo for aneuploidy in women with unexplained RPL, may improve the prognosis for such women. A systematic review that was performed to assess this question concluded that although the miscarriage rates following PGS may be slightly lower, the lack of RCTs, the invasiveness of ART, and the relatively good prognosis of women with unexplained RPL and natural conception renders this treatment inappropriate until further robust data are available.[21] This view is also held by the ESHRE PGD consortium[22] and the practice committees of the ASRM and the Society for Assisted Reproductive Technology.[23]

The Endometrium

Other than looking at the embryo itself as a cause for unexplained RPL, another focus in the recent years has been the endometrium, and its ability to distinguish between good-quality and poor-quality embryos.[24] A preliminary study showed that women with RPL expressed increased levels of proimplantation cytokines, which rendered approximately 40% of them superfertile.[25] The investigators hypothesized that this superfertility disables the natural selection of healthy embryos and allows implantation of poor-quality embryos, which subsequently inevitably leads to pregnancy loss. A subsequent study attempted to investigate this further by looking at endometrial stromal cell migratory activity in response to high-quality and low-quality human embryos.[26] In women with RPL, the migratory activity did not differ between high-quality and low-quality embryos, whereas in the fertile control group the migratory activity was inhibited in low-quality embryos in comparison with high-quality embryos. It is hoped that future studies focusing on the mechanisms by which low-quality embryos inhibit human stromal cell migratory activity will provide further insight into the embryo-endometrial interactions that control implantation and ultimately determine the pregnancy outcome.

Systemic Factors

Other than the embryo-endometrial interactions, a plethora of research has focused on systemic conditions as a possible cause of unexplained RPL. Until these conditions are proved to have a causal effect, most women with these abnormalities may still be diagnosed as having unexplained RPL. Thyroid abnormalities, and particularly thyroid antibodies, have been associated with miscarriage in a recent meta-analysis of evidence,[27] although the treatment with thyroxine has yet to be of proven benefit in the context of unexplained RPL.[28] Polycystic ovary syndrome, insulin resistance, and hyperadrogenemia have all been linked with unexplained RPL,[29] although treatment with insulin-sensitizing agents such as metformin to reduce pregnancy loss remains debatable. A systematic review and meta-analysis showed preconception metformin did not reduce rates of pregnancy loss in women with infertility, whereas small retrospective studies have shown reductions in rates of pregnancy loss in women with previous miscarriages.[30,31] Abnormal immunologic reactions have also been extensively examined with regard to unexplained RPL. Peripheral and uterine natural killer cells have been associated with unexplained RPL in some case-control studies; however, the current evidence does not justify their routine use as prognostic indicators or their subsequent treatment with immunotherapy.[32] Immunologic reaction to male-specific minor histocompatibility H-Y antigens has also been hypothesized as a cause of pregnancy loss in women with secondary unexplained RPL following the birth of a boy.[33] Two studies have indirectly supported this hypothesis by showing that male sex of the first-born child is a strong negative prognostic factor in women with secondary RPL,[34,35] emphasizing the need for further research into this area.

PROGNOSIS OF UNEXPLAINED RECURRENT PREGNANCY LOSS
Traditional View

Traditionally, women with unexplained RPL have been thought to have an excellent prognosis in subsequent pregnancies without the need for any surgical or pharmacologic intervention. This idea has been based predominantly on 3 small nonrandomized trials that have shown reduction in rates of pregnancy loss of up to 50% in women who received psychological supportive care in a dedicated clinic, in comparison with patients who either did not return to the clinic or were looked after in a routine antenatal setting.[12,36] The conclusions drawn from these trials have led to the globally recognized concept of tender love and care (TLC) in the setting of unexplained RPL. However, there were serious limitations in these trials. The first study by the Stray-Pedersens[36] was performed in 1984 at a time when routine investigations such as antiphospholipid screening did not exist. Furthermore, the control group consisted of 24 women who attended a local antenatal care clinic geographically further away from the investigators' dedicated clinic. The second study by Liddell and colleagues[37] in 1991 reported on only 9 women who did not receive psychological supportive care, whereas in the study by Clifford and colleagues[12] in 1997, the control group consisted of 41 women who failed to return to the clinic and had to be contacted by phone or letter for their future outcomes to be established. Despite the limitations of these studies, the concept of psychological supportive care/TLC has been widely accepted and incorporated into various national guidelines.[38,39] However, although TLC broadly consists of serial ultrasonographic scans to confirm viability along with access to specialist counseling, historically it has not been a well-defined entity, and therefore it has been difficult to examine the mechanism through which it operates.[40] A recent survey has attempted to characterize women's preferences for supportive care, and has identified needs such as frequency of ultrasonograms, number of doctors, type of soft skills, and aftercare that women find the most reassuring.[41] It is hoped that future controlled studies will be able to quantify these variables and assess their effect on the pregnancy outcome of women with unexplained RPL.

Novel Views

More recently, it has been proposed that the favorable prognosis in women with unexplained RPL may not be due to psychological supportive care/TLC.[7] It was proposed that because a significant proportion of women with unexplained RPL will be healthy women that have suffered RPL attributable to chance, their prognosis without any intervention will be favorable and similar to that of women in the general population. In analyzing 844 women with untreated unexplained RPL, it was found that the subsequent pregnancy loss of 14% to 26% was almost identical to the 12% to 25% rate of pregnancy loss in the general population for women aged 25 to 39 years. It is therefore concluded that although psychological supportive care/TLC is a commendable and positive experience for women with unexplained RPL, it is unlikely to be the reason why their prognosis in subsequent pregnancies is good.

STRATIFICATION OF WOMEN WITH UNEXPLAINED RECURRENT PREGNANCY LOSS

Although most women with unexplained RPL will have favorable outcomes, a proportion will continue to suffer pregnancy losses, which would imply that they have not suffered their pregnancy losses because of chance and have a genuinely unidentified pathologic cause. Other than the great difficulty the women will have in coming to terms with the condition, these women will be the most difficult to manage from a clinical point of view as there will be no evidence-based treatment to offer. However, such women benefit most from enrolling in well-designed trials investigating novel disorders and treatments.

The key is therefore to identify and distinguish between women with unexplained RPL who have suffered their pregnancy losses by chance alone and women with unexplained RPL and genuine abnormality. It has recently been proposed that these groups can be classified as having type I and type II unexplained RPL, respectively.[7] The characteristics of these 2 groups of women are summarized in **Table 4**.

Table 4				
Characteristics of women with type I and type II unexplained RPL				
		Pregnancy Losses		
	Age	Number	Types	Likely Pathology
Type I	Older	<3	Includes biochemical	Abnormal karyotype of conceptus
Type II	Younger	>3	Clinical only	Remains unidentifiable

Data from Saravelos SH, Li TC. Unexplained recurrent miscarriage: how can we explain it? Hum Rep 2012;27(7):1885.

SUMMARY

Women with unexplained RPL represent a highly heterogeneous group. Some women will have suffered RPL attributable to chance alone, whereas others will have genuine pathologic status that cannot be identified by the current investigative protocols. The definition used to diagnose RPL will significantly affect not only the incidence of women with RPL but also the proportion of women with unexplained RPL. As a result, if women with 2 pregnancy losses and biochemical pregnancy losses are included in the definition, most women may be diagnosed with unexplained RPL and may be entirely healthy. Conversely, if 3 pregnancy losses and clinical pregnancy losses alone are included in the definition, less than one-third of women diagnosed will have suffered RPL because of chance, and therefore the cohort will contain more women with genuine abnormality. Past studies have investigated systemic endocrine and immunologic mechanisms as potential causes of pregnancy loss in unexplained RPL, whereas recent work has focused on spermatozoal, embryonic, and endometrial characteristics to explain the regulation of implantation and subsequent pregnancy loss. Future stratification of women with unexplained RPL, both in the clinical and research context, according to whether they have a high probability of pathologic status, will help select women who are more appropriate for further investigation and potential future treatment.

ACKNOWLEDGMENTS

The authors wish to acknowledge the support from the National Institute for Health Research Imperial Biomedical Research Centre.

REFERENCES

1. Christiansen OB, Nybo Andersen AM, Bosch E, et al. Evidence-based investigations and treatments of recurrent pregnancy loss. Fertil Steril 2005;83(4):821–39.
2. Nybo Andersen AM, Wohlfahrt J, Christens P, et al. Maternal age and fetal loss: population based register linkage study. BMJ 2000;320(7251):1708–12.
3. American Society for Reproductive Medicine. Definitions of infertility and recurrent pregnancy loss. Fertil Steril 2008;90(Suppl 5):S60.
4. Farquharson RG, Jauniaux E, Exalto N. Updated and revised nomenclature for description of early pregnancy events. Hum Rep 2005;20(11):3008–11.
5. Chard T. Frequency of implantation and early pregnancy loss in natural cycles. Baillieres Clin Obstet Gynaecol 1991;5(1):179–89.
6. Roberts CJ. Letter: where have all the conceptions gone? Lancet 1975;1(7907):636.
7. Saravelos SH, Li TC. Unexplained recurrent miscarriage: how can we explain it? Hum Rep 2012;27(7):1882–6.

8. Brigham SA, Conlon C, Farquharson RG. A longitudinal study of pregnancy outcome following idiopathic recurrent miscarriage. Hum Rep 1999;14(11): 2868–71.
9. Hassold T, Chiu D. Maternal age-specific rates of numerical chromosome abnormalities with special reference to trisomy. Hum Genet 1985;70(1):11–7.
10. Regan L, Rai R. Epidemiology and the medical causes of miscarriage. Baillieres Best Pract Res Clin Obstet Gynaecol 2000;14(5):839–54.
11. Li TC, Iqbal T, Anstie B, et al. An analysis of the pattern of pregnancy loss in women with recurrent miscarriage. Fertil Steril 2002;78(5):1100–6.
12. Clifford K, Rai R, Regan L. Future pregnancy outcome in unexplained recurrent first trimester miscarriage. Hum Rep 1997;12(2):387–9.
13. Stephenson MD, Awartani KA, Robinson WP. Cytogenetic analysis of miscarriages from couples with recurrent miscarriage: a case-control study. Hum Rep 2002;17(2):446–51.
14. Rai R, Regan L. Recurrent miscarriage. Lancet 2006;368(9535):601–11.
15. Kaandorp SP, Goddijn M, van der Post JA, et al. Aspirin plus heparin or aspirin alone in women with recurrent miscarriage. N Engl J Med 2010;362(17):1586–96.
16. Ata B, Tan SL, Shehata F, et al. A systematic review of intravenous immunoglobulin for treatment of unexplained recurrent miscarriage. Fertil Steril 2011;95(3): 1080–5.e1–2.
17. Yuan X, Lin HY, Wang Q, et al. Is premature ovarian ageing a cause of unexplained recurrent miscarriage? J Obstet Gynaecol 2012;32(5):464–6.
18. Remohi J, Gallardo E, Levy M, et al. Oocyte donation in women with recurrent pregnancy loss. Hum Rep 1996;11(9):2048–51.
19. Vissenberg R, Goddijn M. Is there a role for assisted reproductive technology in recurrent miscarriage? Semin Reprod Med 2011;29(6):548–56.
20. Robinson L, Gallos ID, Conner SJ, et al. The effect of sperm DNA fragmentation on miscarriage rates: a systematic review and meta-analysis. Hum Rep 2012; 27(10):2908–17.
21. Musters AM, Repping S, Korevaar JC, et al. Pregnancy outcome after preimplantation genetic screening or natural conception in couples with unexplained recurrent miscarriage: a systematic review of the best available evidence. Fertil Steril 2011;95(6):2153–7.e3.
22. Thornhill AR, deDie-Smulders CE, Geraedts JP, et al. ESHRE PGD Consortium 'best practice guidelines for clinical preimplantation genetic diagnosis (PGD) and preimplantation genetic screening (PGS)'. Hum Rep 2005;20(1):35–48.
23. Practice Committee of the American Society for Reproductive Medicine, Practice Committee of the Society for Assisted Reproductive Technology. Preimplantation genetic diagnosis. Fertil Steril 2006;86(5 Suppl 1):S257–8.
24. Teklenburg G, Salker M, Molokhia M, et al. Natural selection of human embryos: decidualizing endometrial stromal cells serve as sensors of embryo quality upon implantation. Plos One 2010;5(4):e10258.
25. Salker M, Teklenburg G, Molokhia M, et al. Natural selection of human embryos: impaired decidualization of endometrium disables embryo-maternal interactions and causes recurrent pregnancy loss. Plos One 2010;5(4):e10287.
26. Weimar CH, Kavelaars A, Brosens JJ, et al. Endometrial stromal cells of women with recurrent miscarriage fail to discriminate between high- and low-quality human embryos. Plos One 2012;7(7):e41424.
27. Thangaratinam S, Tan A, Knox E, et al. Association between thyroid autoantibodies and miscarriage and preterm birth: meta-analysis of evidence. BMJ 2011;342:d2616.

28. Yan J, Sripada S, Saravelos SH, et al. Thyroid peroxidase antibody in women with unexplained recurrent miscarriage: prevalence, prognostic value, and response to empirical thyroxine therapy. Fertil Steril 2012;98(2):378–82.

29. Smith ML, Schust DJ. Endocrinology and recurrent early pregnancy loss. Semin Reprod Med 2011;29(6):482–90.

30. Jakubowicz DJ, Iuorno MJ, Jakubowicz S, et al. Effects of metformin on early pregnancy loss in the polycystic ovary syndrome. J Clin Endocrinol Metab 2002;87(2):524–9.

31. Glueck CJ, Phillips H, Cameron D, et al. Continuing metformin throughout pregnancy in women with polycystic ovary syndrome appears to safely reduce first-trimester spontaneous abortion: a pilot study. Fertil Steril 2001;75(1):46–52.

32. Tang AW, Alfirevic Z, Quenby S. Natural killer cells and pregnancy outcomes in women with recurrent miscarriage and infertility: a systematic review. Hum Rep 2011;26(8):1971–80.

33. Nielsen HS. Secondary recurrent miscarriage and H-Y immunity. Hum Reprod Update 2011;17(4):558–74.

34. Nielsen HS, Andersen AM, Kolte AM, et al. A firstborn boy is suggestive of a strong prognostic factor in secondary recurrent miscarriage: a confirmatory study. Fertil Steril 2008;89(4):907–11.

35. Christiansen OB, Pedersen B, Nielsen HS, et al. Impact of the sex of first child on the prognosis in secondary recurrent miscarriage. Hum Rep 2004;19(12):2946–51.

36. Stray-Pedersen B, Stray-Pedersen S. Etiologic factors and subsequent reproductive performance in 195 couples with a prior history of habitual abortion. Am J Obstet Gynecol 1984;148(2):140–6.

37. Liddell HS, Pattison NS, Zanderigo A. Recurrent miscarriage—outcome after supportive care in early pregnancy. Aust N Z J Obstet Gynaecol 1991;31(4):320–2.

38. American College of Obstetricians and Gynecologists. ACOG practice bulletin. Management of recurrent pregnancy loss. Number 24, February 2001. (Replaces Technical Bulletin Number 212, September 1995). American College of Obstetricians and Gynecologists. Int J Gynaecol Obstet 2002;78(2):179–90.

39. Royal College of Obstetricians and Gynaecologists. Green top guideline No. 17. The investigation and treatment of couples with recurrent first trimester miscarriage and second trimester miscarriage. RCOG. 2011.

40. Li TC, Makris M, Tomsu M, et al. Recurrent miscarriage: aetiology, management and prognosis. Hum Reprod Update 2002;8(5):463–81.

41. Musters AM, Koot YE, van den Boogaard NM, et al. Supportive care for women with recurrent miscarriage: a survey to quantify women's preferences. Hum Rep 2013;28(2):398–405.

Index

Note: Page numbers of article titles are in **boldface** type.

A

Acquired thrombophilias, 137
Adhesion(s)
   intrauterine
      RPL related to, 6
   RPL related to, 69–73
      causes of, 69–72
      characteristics of, 69
      classification of, 69
      first-trimester pregnancy loss due to, 72
      prevalence of, 72
      treatment of, 72–73
Age
   maternal
      as factor in unexplained RPL, 159
Alcohol consumption
   RPL related to, 13
Amniocentesis
   in reproductive medicine, 45–46
Aneuploidy
   basics of, 44–45
   recurrent
      RPL related to, 12
Antenatal genetic testing
   in reproductive medicine, 43–46
      amniocentesis, 45–46
      aneuploidy, 44–45
      cell-free fetal DNA evaluation, 46
      CVS, 45–46
Antibody(ies)
   antiphospholipid. *See* Antiphospholipid antibody(ies) (aPLs)
Antinuclear antibodies
   RPL related to, 10–11
Antiphospholipid antibody(ies) (aPLs)
   thrombosis and, 121–122
Antiphospholipid antibody syndrome (APS), **113–132**
   defective placentation and, 122
   diagnosis of, 114–118
      clinical criteria in, 114–116
      laboratory criteria in, 117–118
   introduction, 113–114
   lifelong consequences of, 126

Obstet Gynecol Clin N Am 41 (2014) 167–176
http://dx.doi.org/10.1016/S0889-8545(13)00123-X
0889-8545/14/$ – see front matter © 2014 Elsevier Inc. All rights reserved.

obgyn.theclinics.com

Antiphospholipid (*continued*)
    local inflammatory events and, 122–123
    management of
        heparin in, 123
        in pregnancy, 123–125
            antepartum surveillance, 125
            overview of, 123–124
            unfractionated heparin *vs.* LMWH, 124–125
    MTL related to, 90
        treatment of, 90
    obstetric complications of, 118–120
    pathophysiology of, 120–123
    postpregnancy considerations, 126
    RPL related to, 9–10, 118–120
    severe placental insufficiency related to, 120
Antithrombin deficiency
    inherited thrombophilias related to, 136–137
aPLs. *See* Antiphospholipid antibody(ies) (aPLs)
APS. *See* Antiphospholipid antibody syndrome (APS)
Arcuate uterus, 61
    metroplasty for, 68

B

Bicornuate uterus, 59, 60
    metroplasty for, 68

C

Caffeine intake
    RPL related to, 13
Cell-free fetal DNA evaluation
    in reproductive medicine, 46
Cervical cerclage
    for RPL related to uterine anomalies, 68–69
Cervical occlusion
    in cervical weakness–related MTL management, 95–96
Cervical weakness
    MTL related to, 93–98. *See also* Mid-trimester pregnancy loss (MTL), cervical weakness
        and
Cervix
    incompetent
        RPL related to, 7
Chorionic villus sampling (CVS)
    in reproductive medicine, 45–46
Chromosomal disorders
    parental
        RPL related to, 11–12
Cigarette smoking
    RPL related to, 13
Congenital malformations

RPL related to, 5–6
CVS. *See* Chorionic villus sampling (CVS)

D

DES. *See* Diethylstilbestrol (DES)
Didelphic uterus, 59, 60
    metroplasty for, 68
Diethylstilbestrol (DES) drug-related uterus, 61

E

Embryo(s)
    euploid
        developmental errors in
            RPL related to, 12
Endocrine system
    in RPL, **103–112**. *See also* Recurrent pregnancy loss (RPL), endocrine basis for
Environmental factors
    uterine anomalies related to
        RPL due to, 61
Environmental toxins
    RPL related to, 12–13
Euploid embryos
    developmental errors in
        RPL related to, 12

F

Factor V Leiden
    inherited thrombophilias related to, 135–136
Fibroid(s)
    RPL related to, 73–76
        causes of, 74
        characteristics of, 73–74
        classification of, 73–74
        first-trimester pregnancy loss due to, 75
        prevalence of, 74–75
        treatment of, 75–76
First-trimester pregnancy loss
    adhesions and, 72
    fibroids and, 75
    polyps and, 77
    uterine anomalies and, 64–67

G

Genetic(s)
    in reproductive medicine, **41–55**
        evolving role of, **41–55**
        genetic analysis following fetal demise, 52

Genetic(s) (*continued*)
    introduction, 42
    preconception genetic testing, 42–43
    preimplantation genetic testing, 46–52
  RPL related to, 11–12
  uterine anomalies related to
    RPL due to, 62
Genetic testing
  antenatal, 43–46
  preconception, 42–43
Glucose metabolism
  abnormal
    RPL related to, 8

H

Heparin
  in APS management, 123
  low-molecular-weight
    in APS management in pregnancy
      vs. unfractionated heparin, 124–125
  unfractionated
    in APS management in pregnancy
      vs. LMWH, 124–125
Hyperprolactinemia
  RPL related to, 8
Hypothyroidism
  untreated
    RPL related to, 8

I

Immunologic disorders
  RPL related to, 9
Immunotherapy
  RPL related to, 10
Incompetent cervix
  RPL related to, 7
Infection(s)
  MTL related to, 90–92
Inherited thrombophilias, **133–144**
  antithrombin deficiency and, 136–137
  combined defects, 137
  discussion, 140–141
  factor V Leiden and, 135–136
  future directions in, 141–142
  introduction, 133–134
  MTHFR and, 137
  overview of, 134–135
  protein C deficiency and, 136
  protein S deficiency and, 136
  prothrombin and, 136

research related to, 141–142
    testing criteria for, 139–140
    treatment of, 138–141
        physician practice patterns in, 139–140
Intrauterine adhesions
    RPL related to, 6
Intrauterine masses
    RPL related to, 6–7
Ionizing radiation
    RPL related to, 13

L

Lifestyle issues
    RPL related to, 12–13
LMWH. *See* Low-molecular-weight heparin (LMWH)
Low-molecular-weight heparin (LMWH)
    in APS management in pregnancy
        vs. unfractionated heparin, 124–125
Luteal phase defect
    RPL related to, 104–105
Luteal phase deficiency
    RPL related to, 7

M

Mass(es)
    intrauterine
        RPL related to, 6–7
Maternal age
    as factor in unexplained RPL, 159
Methylene tetrahydrofolate reductase (MTHFR)
    inherited thrombophilias related to, 137
Metroplasty
    for RPL-related to uterine anomalies, 68
Microbiologic agents
    RPL related to, 11
Mid-trimester pregnancy loss (MTL), **87–102**
    APS and, 90
    cervical weakness and, 93–98
        described, 93–94
        management of, 94–98
            cervical occlusion in, 95–96
            progesterone in, 94–95
            TAC in, 96–98
            TVC in, 95
            ultrasound assessment in, 94
    classification of, 87
    defined, 87
    infection and, 90–92
    introduction, 87–88

Mid-trimester (*continued*)
  pathology associated with, 90
  screening protocol for, 88–90
  treatment of, 90
  uterine anomalies and, 92–93
Miscarriage(s)
  causes of
    mechanisms of, 67
  described, 145
  recurrent. *See* Recurrent miscarriage(s) (RMs)
  unexplained RPL and, 158
MTHFR. *See* Methylene tetrahydrofolate reductase (MTHFR)
MTL. *See* Mid-trimester pregnancy loss (MTL)
Müllerian duct(s)
  differentiation of
    defects in, 61
  fusion of
    defects in, 59, 60
  1
    defects in formation of, 59

  O

Obesity
  RPL related to, 13
Ovarian reserve
  diminished
    RPL related to, 8–9

  P

Parental chromosomal disorders
  RPL related to, 11–12
PCOS. *See* Polycystic ovarian syndrome (PCOS)
PGS. *See* Preimplantation genetic screening (PGS)
Placental insufficiency
  severe
    RPL related to, 120
Polycystic ovarian syndrome (PCOS)
  RPL related to, 108–109
Polyp(s)
  RPL related to, 77–78
Preconception genetic testing
  in reproductive medicine, 42–43
Pregnancy
  APS in
    management of, 123–125. *See also* Antiphospholipid antibody syndrome (APS),
      management of, in pregnancy
Pregnancy loss
  causes of
    mechanisms of, 67

defined, 2
early. *See also* Recurrent pregnancy loss (RPL)
    management of, **1–18**
        introduction, 1–2
first-trimester
    adhesions and, 72
    fibroids and, 75
    polyps and, 77
    uterine anomalies and, 64–67
mid-trimester, **87–102**. *See also* Mid-trimester pregnancy loss (MTL)
Preimplantation genetic diagnosis
    in reproductive medicine, 47–48
Preimplantation genetic screening (PGS)
    in reproductive medicine, 48–51
        clinical application of, 51
        limitations of, 51–52
Preimplantation genetic testing
    in reproductive medicine, 46–52
        diagnosis-related, 47–48
        PGS, 48–51
    in RPL detection, 12
Progesterone
    in cervical weakness–related MTL management, 94–95
Protein C deficiency
    inherited thrombophilias related to, 136
Protein S deficiency
    inherited thrombophilias related to, 136
Prothrombin
    inherited thrombophilias related to, 136

R

Radiation
    ionizing
        RPL related to, 13
Randomized controlled trials (RCTs)
    in RPL research, 33–35
RCTs. *See* Randomized controlled trials (RCTs)
Recurrent aneuploidy
    RPL related to, 12
Recurrent miscarriage(s) (RMs)
    described, 145
    guidelines related to, 146–147
Recurrent miscarriage clinics, **145–155**
    doctor preferences, 150–151
    introduction, 145–146
    logistic requirements for, 147–150
        equipment, 148–149
        laboratory services, 149
        location, 147
        record keeping, 149

Recurrent (*continued*)
    rooms, 147
    staffing, 147
  one-stop, 149–150
  patient preferences, 152–153
  recommendations, 153
Recurrent pregnancy loss (RPL)
  APS and, 9–10, 118–120
  causes of, 2–3, 57
    anatomic, 5–7
    autoimmune/thrombotic factors, 9–11
    endocrinologic, 7–9
    environmental toxins, 12–13
    genetic factors, 11–12
    lifestyle issues, 12–13
  chance as factor in, 160
  defined, 2, 157–158
    controversies related to, 20–21
  diagnosis of, 3–5
  endocrine basis for, **103–112**
    luteal phase defect, 104–105
    PCOS, 108–109
    thyroid disease, 105–108
  introduction, 1–2
  outcome of, 13–14
  prevalence of, 2
  research methodology in, **19–39**
    case-control studies, 22–29
      flaws in estimating risk factors, 24–28
      flaws in sampling of patients and controls, 22–24
      interpretation, 29
      lack of protocol data or priory hypothesis, 28–29
      multiple testing, 29
    cohort studies, 29–32
      cohorts estimating live births per time unit, 32
      concurrent *vs.* nonconcurrent cohorts, 30
      nonrandom misclassification, 30–32
    introduction, 19–20
    research studies, 21–22
    treatment trials, 32–36
      historical controls, 32–33
      RCTs, 33–35
      systematic reviews, 35–36
  risk factors for, 2
  treatment of, 3–5
  unexplained, **157–166**. *See also* Unexplained recurrent pregnancy loss (RPL)
  uterine anomalies and, **57–86**. *See also* Uterine anomalies, RPL related to
Reproductive medicine
  genetics in
    evolving role of, **41–55**. *See also* Genetic(s), in reproductive medicine
RM. *See* Recurrent miscarriage(s) (RMs)

S

Septate uterus, 61
  metroplasty for, 68
Septum
  regression of
    defects in, 61
Severe placental insufficiency
  RPL related to, 120
Single-gene disorders
  in reproductive medicine, 47–48
Smoking
  RPL related to, 13
Structural chromosome aberrations
  in reproductive medicine, 48

T

TAC. *See* Transabdominal cerclage (TAC)
Thrombophilia(s)
  acquired, 137
  inherited, **133–144**. *See also* Inherited thrombophilias
Thrombotic disorders
  RPL related to, 11
Thyroid disease
  RPL related to, 105–108
Toxin(s)
  environmental
    RPL related to, 12–13
Transabdominal cerclage (TAC)
  in cervical weakness–related MTL management, 96–98
    research evidence for, 96–98
Transvaginal cervical cerclage (TVC)
  in cervical weakness–related MTL management, 95
TVC. *See* Transvaginal cervical cerclage (TVC)

U

Ultrasound
  in cervical weakness–related MTL management, 94
Unexplained recurrent pregnancy loss (RPL), **157–166**
  causes of, 160–162
  defined, 157–158
  incidence of, 159–160
  maternal age as factor in, 159
  miscarriages suffered due to, 158
  prevalence of, 160
  prognosis of, 162–163
  stratification of women with, 163–164
Unfractionated heparin
  in APS management in pregnancy
    vs. LMWH, 124–125

Unicornuate uterus, 59
    metroplasty for, 68
Uterine anomalies
    congenital, 59–61
        classification and embryology of, 59–61
    MTL related to, 92–93
    RPL related to, **57–86**
        acquired, 69–78
        adhesions, 69–73
        causes of, 61–62
        congenital, 64–67
        diagnosis of
            imaging in, 58
        fibroids, 73–76
        introduction, 57
        polyps, 77–78
        prevalence of, 62–64
        treatment of, 68–69
Uterus
    arcuate, 61
        metroplasty for, 68
    bicornuate, 59, 60
        metroplasty for, 68
    DES drug-related, 61
    didelphic, 59, 60
        metroplasty for, 68
    embryology of, 58
    septate, 61
        metroplasty for, 68
    unicornuate, 59
        metroplasty for, 68

Moving?

Make sure your subscription moves with you!

To notify us of your new address, find your **Clinics Account Number** (located on your mailing label above your name), and contact customer service at:

Email: journalscustomerservice-usa@elsevier.com

800-654-2452 (subscribers in the U.S. & Canada)
314-447-8871 (subscribers outside of the U.S. & Canada)

Fax number: 314-447-8029

Elsevier Health Sciences Division
Subscription Customer Service
3251 Riverport Lane
Maryland Heights, MO 63043

*To ensure uninterrupted delivery of your subscription, please notify us at least 4 weeks in advance of move.

Printed and bound by CPI Group (UK) Ltd, Croydon, CR0 4YY

03/10/2024

01040485-0013